Healing
Childhood Ear Infections

Healing
Childhood Ear Infections

Prevention, Home Care,
and Alternative Treatment

Dr. Michael A. Schmidt

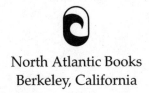

North Atlantic Books
Berkeley, California

Homeopathic Educational Services
Berkeley, California

Healing Childhood Ear Infections:
Prevention, Home Care, and Alternative Treatment

Published by

North Atlantic Books   Homeopathic Educational Services
P.O. Box 12327   2124 Kittredge Street
Berkeley, California 94712   Berkeley, California 94704

Cover photo: Jacob Gregory Ullman, son of Dana and Clare Ullman
Cover and book design by Paula Morrison
Printed in the United States of America

Distributed to the book trade by Publishers Group West

This book discusses the problem of childhood ear infections. It has been written as an educational guide and reference for both laypersons and health care professionals, but it is not intended to replace the services of a physician. Treatment of any illness must be supervised by a licensed health care professional. The author and publisher disclaim all responsibility arising from any adverse effects or results that might occur as a result of the application of any of the information contained in this book. Accordingly, either you or the professional who examines and treats you must take full responsibility for the uses made of this book. Before undertaking any of the self-care treatments described in this book it is advisable to consult your health care professional.

Healing Childhood Ear Infections: Prevention, Home Care, and Alternative Treatment is sponsored by the Society for the Study of Native Arts and Sciences, a nonprofit educational corporation whose goals are to develop an educational and crosscultural perspective linking various scientific, social, and artistic fields; to nurture a holistic view of arts, sciences, humanities, and healing; and to publish and distribute literature on the relationship of mind, body, and nature.

Library of Congress Cataloging-in-Publication Data

Schmidt, Michael A., 1958–
    Healing childhood ear infections : prevention, home care, and
alternative treatment / Michael A. Schmidt. —2nd edition.
       p.   cm
    Previous ed. published as Childhood ear infections.
    Includes index.
    ISBN -1-55643-216-X
    1. Otitis media in children.   2. Otitis media in children—
Alternative treatment.   I. Schmidt, Michael A., 1958–   Childhood
ear infections.   II. Title.
RF225.S36   1996
618.92'09784— dc20   95-53679
                                                  CIP

2   3   4   5   6   7/00   99   98   97   96

Acknowledgments

I am deeply grateful to the pioneering spirits upon whose work I have drawn to synthesize my ideas about the treatment of illness.

I am grateful to my dear colleague David Eisenberg, M.D., of Harvard Medical School for his grace, vision, and insight; for the vigilant search for truth that has been the hallmark of Jack Paradise, M.D. of the University of Pittsburgh; for the valuable summaries, insights, and considerable determination of Erdem Cantekin, Ph.D. of the University of Pittsburgh.

I am grateful to Doris Rapp, M.D., who is truly a jewel of a human being, a delightful soul, and gifted doctor; to William Crook, M.D. and his unwavering pursuit over many decades to help children and inform the public; to George Shambaugh, M.D. who became a standard-bearer for all who strove to look deeper into the mysteries of childhood illness.

I am grateful to Jan Thatcher Adams, M.D. of the University of Minnesota Medical School, who is a model of compassion, wisdom, and thoughtfulness in a physician.

I am grateful to my friend and colleague Jeffrey Bland, Ph.D. He has truly helped raise the level of sophistication of nutrition and preventive medicine to where it stands today.

I am grateful to the editors of the Journal of Chinese Medicine and Dr. Julian Scott for granting me liberal use of their material on pediatric acupuncture. To Martha Benedict for her time and valuable insights into the management of otitis media. To Anastacia White for her contribution on Chinese herbal medicine. To Dr. Stephen Messer for the use of his graphics on homeopathic medicine. To the Project on Government Oversight for their executive summary on antibiotic use. To Joan Fallon, D.C. for use of her tympanographic studies on children and for her devotion to helping people.

I am grateful to my past patients—both children and adults—who challenged me to become a good diagnostician, a compassionate listener, and to learn more.

I am grateful to Ric Alexander and Paula Morrison for weaving the considerable changes into this new edition.

A special thanks to my wife Julie, who endured long hours of editing and sat through endless jargon-filled sessions as I sifted through my ideas. A thanks to my boys, who are a constant source of inspiration, humor, and learning.

Contents

Figures

Foreword

As a pediatric allergist, I personally have seen many infants and children who have had recurrent ear infections secondary to their milk allergies. As Dr. Schmidt so ably describes and explains, this is certainly one of the most common unsuspected causes of this problem. Many do not realize that any dairy product can cause this type of difficulty. As affected children become older and even when they become adults, they often love or hate all dairy products or they crave cheese but refuse to drink milk. These typical strong preferences frequently suggest that any form of dairy is a problem. If a child (or adult) couldn't care less about eating dairy products, then it is less likely that this is a consideration.

Many infants and young children have a typical pattern. They have one ear infection after another, and then one course of antibiotic after another. This leads to an overgrowth of yeast and only temporary relief of the ear complaints. Ultimately, many of these children have repeated doctor or emergency visits, constant or prophylactic antibiotics, and then some form of surgery such as eartubes or adenoid removal. Needless to say, if there is an easy, better, and safer way to more effectively relieve these problems, it should be seriously considered by those parents who have noticed this sequence of events. *Healing Childhood Ear Infections* provides the type of insight that parents need to understand how to approach this type of problem. This book tells you:

- What you wish you knew, before the previous few ear infections.

- Why typical ear infection treatment might not help.

- What can happen if it isn't appropriately treated.

- What can be done to prevent the typical recurrence of ear infections in young children.

- Which alternative forms of treatment are available.

- How effective they are.

As with most medical problems, another trip to the medicine cabinet is often only one more temporary fix. Sometimes a book such as this one provides the bottom line challenge, which is to find out what causes a medical problem. Why does it occur on a specific day or at a particular time? These are the types of questions that Dr. Schmidt addresses in this book. For example, is it an allergy to either breast-milk or formula that is causing an infant's nose tissues to swell so that the opening to the area between the eardrum and nose is blocked? If this is the cause, then the treatment is not another course of the right antibiotic or to put a small, hollow, tiny tube through the eardrum. The answer is to stop the milk, or treat the milk sensitivity so that the nose doesn't swell. If this is done, the sinuses don't become blocked and the middle ear functions normally. The key question to repeatedly ask is "why?" What did my child, eat, smell, or touch that could have caused this present problem. Was it due to something inside, outside, a food, or a chemical?

One of the difficulties with food-related ear problems is the fact that there is typically a delay in the onset of symptoms. If you are drinking milk and that causes an allergy, there can be a day or so between the time a child drinks milk and the time the ear infection becomes apparent. For example, milk causes some children to develop part or all of these complaints. Some children become stuffy, repeatedly clear their throats, make clucking sounds, and act irritable or hyperactive within an hour after drinking milk. That night they may cry because of asthma or leg aches and then wet the bed. The next day they might have difficulty hearing and the following day have a full blown ear infection. Even though this type of pattern is repeated over and over, the sequence is frequently not recognized.

Ear problems related to dust, molds, and exposure to natural gas or tobacco similarly can be delayed for a day or two. Unlike allergies due to sugar or red food dyes, which so commonly cause a bout of hyperactivity or unprovoked and unacceptable behavior in less than an hour, it takes a while for fluid to accumulate between the nose and the eardrum.

In this book, Dr. Schmidt tells you how to spot these types of relationships and what parents must think about. Additional common sense knowledge is certainly an asset in today's fast-paced society. Many times caring parents can find answers that others have repeatedly missed because of the type of information that is discussed in this book. The more you understand about what causes recurrent ear or sinus problems, the sooner you can take measures to eliminate the problem, not only in your child, but, also, in yourself.

Antibiotics are certainly helpful—but you must understand that they are a double-edged sword that should not be used unless absolutely necessary. Parents walk a fine line trying to make decisions in relation to health problems in their children. In general, as indicated in this book, there are other approaches that, at times, are surprisingly effective. At one point I laughed when a particular mother said that homeopathic remedies could effectively eliminate ear problems. I recall vividly when she came into my office and asked me to check her child's ears. The eardrums were fiery red. I strongly suggested that she start an antibiotic immediately. I told her that if this was not done, I would be concerned about how that youngster would be that evening and the next morning. This mother very adamantly refused and said that she would not give the antibiotics, and she was going to try homeopathic remedies instead. I warned her it was imperative that she start the antibiotic as soon as possible, and to forget the homeopathic remedies. The next morning she returned to the office. I looked into the child's ears and I was truly surprised to see that the ear drums appeared to be almost normal. I told her that I was pleased that she had decided to fill the antibiotic prescription. She informed me that she had only treated the child with homeopathic remedies. At that time I realized that, once again, we doctors have much to learn. There are different ways to approach medical problems and we must continually seek those that are faster, easier, more effective, and less expensive. There is no doubt in my mind that some children's ear problems can be controlled very effectively with certain types of herbs and homeopathic remedies. This book discusses the specifics of how to make such decisions: when and what to use. With this knowledge you can not only attempt to initially treat an infection but you can learn how to prevent future episodes. If it isn't helpful within a short period of time you should definitely check with your physician.

Some parents believe that it is easier and faster to treat their child with an antibiotic rather than try to figure out why they have recurrent infections. Busy single mothers already have more to do than they can handle, and some are desperate to find anything that will stop the infections. Many know that antibiotics may be easier initially, but the nights when your child cries in pain, and the problems that are created by the repeated or prolonged, intermittent or constant, use of antibiotics cannot be discounted. The knowledge that is conveyed in this book will certainly help you to recognize that although antibiotics are helpful, you need to consider the positive and negative in relation to any form of drug therapy.

This is a balanced book that presents both sides of the issues. If your doctor is skeptical, you might loan or give him a copy of this book. Most doctors would be pleased to look it over and surprised by some of the convincing evidence and material that is presented in the book.

This kind of insight and knowledge will enable you to provide your child with a happier, healthier life. The fundamental principles that are explained in this book apply to more than the present ear infections. Other chronic illnesses that are so commonly seen in young children with allergies or environmental illness have the same basic relation to diet and stress that ear infections do. Dr. Schmidt has written a balanced, informative, and practical presentation of the facts and fallacies of ear infections. This information will help your child and your family for many years. Don't loan it to your neighbor, because you might never see it again.

—Doris J. Rapp, M.D.
Author of *Is This Your Child?* and *Sick Schools, Sick Kids, Sick Teachers*

Introduction

Ear infections are the number-one reason parents bring their children to the doctor. Over the last ten years, the number of children who get earaches has risen sharply. As a parent and a doctor, I am concerned about the high numbers of children affected by this illness and about what conventional medicine has to offer. Certainly, we all know there are children with ear infections who have been benefited by antibiotics and tubes. But, we also know those who have not been helped. Indeed, there are even children who have been hurt by these forms of treatment.

Because of this, I have spent considerable time investigating the current medical methods of treatment and the alternatives that are available. One would not know from the popular press that doctors are not wholly successful at treating ear infections in children. It is surprising that the media has not addressed this. But there is now evidence that demands we take a new look at an old and growing problem. Consider these findings:

- When antibiotics are used at the beginning of an acute middle ear infection, the frequency of recurrent infections may be almost three times greater than if antibiotics are delayed or not used.[1]

- Antibiotics have been shown not to affect the outcome of acute middle ear infection with regard to pain, fever, hearing, and healing time.[2]

- There appears to be little difference in outcome of middle ear infections treated with a three-day course of antibiotic when compared with those treated with the typical ten-day course of antibiotic.[3]

- Eardrum scarring with membrane thickening has been found to occur in over 40 percent of children receiving tubes compared with zero percent in those not receiving tubes.[4]

- Many cases of chronic middle ear infection, even those with eardrum perforation, are due to allergy.[5]

- In up to 70 percent of children with middle ear "infection" who do not respond to antibiotics, the middle ear fluid contains no harmful bacteria.[6]

- Zinc deficient children suffer from more ear infections than those with normal zinc status. There is evidence that nutrition may play a crucial role in the prevention and treatment of recurrent ear infections.[7]

In this book, I examine the scope of the ear infection problem. I take a careful look at the current methods of treatment. Antibiotics and tubes are discussed in depth because they are not, however, without risk or side effect. I take a new look at causes of ear infections and present a discussion of diet and nutrition that has significant implications. The home care and prevention chapters are valuable to parents because of the practical information they contain. What may ultimately be the most useful is the section on alternative treatment, in which I describe the methods used by holistic doctors to treat earaches.

My purpose is not to condemn conventional medicine, since I recognize its inherent value and tremendous contributions. However, we must realize that medicine is a collaborative effort—one that embraces the useful features of all healing systems. It is my hope that the medicine of the twenty-first century will be a mixture of the science of medicine and the art of healing, that will be a way of viewing the patient as a whole, while understanding the function of his parts. It is only after such a synthesis that we can say our system of healing has evolved to truly serve the needs of our children and ourselves.

—Michael A. Schmidt, D.C., C.C.N., C.N.S.

Chapter 1

The Scope
of the Problem

The treatment of recurrent otitis media remains an unresolved problem.[1]

Leon Eisenberg, M.D.

Tiffany was just nine months old when she experienced her first ear infection. It began with sleepless nights, irritability, and fussiness at dinner time. Before long it was obvious that she was ill and needed attention. Her parents took her to the pediatrician. Diagnosis—acute otitis media. Tiffany was treated with antibiotics. Within two weeks, her ears improved, but within four weeks, the ear infection had returned.

Back to the pediatrician. Tiffany's doctor again prescribed antibiotics. After two weeks, she showed improvement. But the ear infection returned within four weeks. The cycle continued. By the time Tiffany was twenty-one months old, she had received antibiotics on eleven separate occasions—all to no avail. Tiffany's parents were exhausted and frustrated. They felt helpless at their inability to do anything for their daughter. The effects of repeated antibiotics concerned them. When Tiffany was two and a half years old, her parents agreed to have tubes put in her ears.

The tubes seemed to help. At the beginning, Tiffany could hear somewhat better and the earaches subsided. Gradually, fluid returned and hearing started to diminish. Tiffany was weak, sickly, and irritable. The cycle was starting again.

Ear infections ... antibiotics ... more ear infections ... more antibiotics ... ear infections ... antibiotics. This is the recurring theme for millions of infants and toddlers each year. For many children with recurrent earaches, tubes are the ultimate fate. Yet, in spite of repeated antibiotics and tubes, many children continue to have problems until they are six or seven years old—an age when earaches subside naturally. Tiffany was headed in this direction, but her parents chose a different course.

When Tiffany was four, her parents had grown weary of the unsuccessful attempts to cure her earaches. On the recommendation of a friend, Tiffany's parents took her to a doctor who used natural methods to care for earaches. The new doctor explained that Tiffany had dietary and nutritional problems that previous doctors had not addressed. Tiffany was placed on a diet free of dairy products, eggs, and sulfites—foods to which she tested sensitive. The doctor also prescribed specific nutrients and homeopathic medicines. Within one month of beginning this program, her middle ear effusion cleared. Within two months, her ears had recovered fully. Today, Tiffany is a successful college student. The ear infection she had at age four was her last. She has completely recovered from the hearing problems she suffered as a child and is on the Dean's List. (See chapter 6 for additional details about Tiffany's tubes.)

Tiffany's recovery was swift. Not all ear infections managed in this way improve so quickly. But this case illustrates the value of using natural forms of healing for childhood illness. Tiffany's case is just one of many cases of childhood ear infections treated successfully by doctors around the world using natural methods.

In this book, we'll explore a variety of natural healing methods that are used to care for earaches, along with valuable tips about prevention and home care. Before moving on to this discussion, it is important that you understand some basic things about childhood ear infections—what they are, how they're treated, who's at risk, and complications.

Otitis media, or middle ear inflammation, is the number-one childhood health problem in America. In one survey, it was found to be the most frequently diagnosed illness and the most frequent reason, after well-baby and child care, for visits to a doctor.[2] The diagnosis and treatment of middle ear problems accounts for roughly one-third of all pediatric visits,[3] comprising roughly 30 million visits to the doctor per year.[4] The overall cost of diagnosis and treatment now exceeds 4 billion dollars annually.[5]

For many children, earaches begin in infancy. By the age of three, over two-thirds of all children have had one or more episodes of acute otitis media, including 33 percent who have had three or more episodes.[6] Nearly all children affected continue to have problems until the age of six or seven. Otitis media does not become rare until after age 10,[7] and persists in some children beyond 15 years of age. Boys appear to be affected more often than girls in the younger age groups, while the trend reverses in older children.[8]

In spite of vast increases in the pediatric use of antibiotics, the incidence of otitis media has risen sharply. Most recent evidence shows that since 1975, the number of patient visits has increased almost 150 percent, and the annual rate has more than doubled. The rate in children under two has increased 224 percent.[9] This substantial increase in otitis media has been attributed to everything from increased doctor awareness to improved diagnostic abilities. There are even those who contend that the incidence of otitis media has increased, in part, because of the widespread use of antibiotic drugs.[10] To a degree, any of the above explanations may have merit. However, there are additional factors that have emerged during the past several decades that increase a child's susceptibility to illness such as otitis media. These will be explored in later chapters.

What Is an Earache?

An earache can develop when the tissue lining the middle ear or eustachian tube swells (See figure 1-a.). As the membranes swell, the opening of the eustachian tube gradually becomes obstructed, thereby preventing the middle ear from draining properly. As inflammation of the middle ear builds, the production of fluid increases. In some cases bacteria contribute to the ongoing inflam-

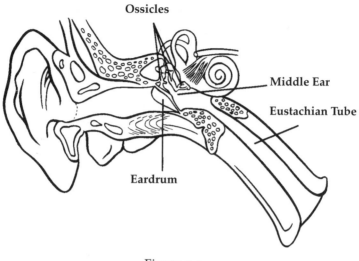

Figure 1-a
Structures of the Ear

mation, while in others the inflammatory response occurs for different reasons.

The congestion within the middle ear causes pressure to be exerted on the eardrum and the sensitive structures that lie within (and near) the middle ear chamber. The pressure exerted on the eardrum can produce one of the most painful sensations your child will ever experience. When the eustachian tube is blocked, there is no way to alter the pressure in the middle ear. In some cases, the eardrum ruptures and fluid drains out, which reduces the pressure. In others, the inflammation subsides and the eustachian tube opens, allowing drainage of fluid. Sometimes treatment is required to encourage proper function of the eustachian tube and reduced production of fluid in the middle ear.

Signs and Symptoms

It may be surprising to know that many instances of otitis media occur with a relative absence of symptoms. Your child may act and hear normally and experience no pain. Yet if the doctor examined the eardrum during a routine physical or for another reason, he may see fluid behind the eardrum. Fluid may even drain from the ear with no other evidence that the child is having problems. Chronic ear infections often occur with little pain. Acute ear infections can be severely painful. In general, pain is one of the most common signs of middle ear problems.

One of the first indicators of a middle ear problem is a change in behavior or sleep habits. This is not specific, however, and could suggest any number of other problems. A child may pull or tug at the ear or frequently poke his finger into the ear canal. This also might indicate itchiness in the ear or a foreign object lodged in the canal. An abrupt or temporary change in hearing acuity may signal a middle ear problem as well.

Older children who can better communicate their feelings might complain of a plugged, blocked, or pressure sensation in the middle ear. Buzzing or ringing sensations may occur.

Symptoms of acute earaches commonly include (although all may not be present in a given child):

- Ear pain.

- Fever.

- Drainage from the ear.

- Sleeplessness.

- Irritability.

- Change in eating habits.

- Change in hearing.

- Refusal to nurse on one side.

- Nasal obstruction or discharge.

In cases of chronic earache, the most notable symptom might be diminished hearing. Behavior changes are also common.

How the Doctor Diagnoses an Ear Infection

The most common method used by all doctors is visual inspection of the eardrum using an otoscope. The otoscope is the familiar hand-held device you've seen the doctor use when looking in your child's ears. When looking in the ear, the appearance of the eardrum is the most important sign. The eardrum has several characteristic land-marks. If any of these land marks have changed in appearance, it may suggest a problem in the middle ear.

Since the eardrum is somewhat transparent, it is possible to see behind it to a limited degree. Behind the eardrum the doctor might observe an arrangement of large or small bubbles—suggesting fluid in the middle ear—or a fluid line. This fluid line will often change position when the child tips her head forward or backward (just as if you had taken a glass full of water and tipped it back and forth).

The eardrum is normally pearly-grey and shiny. If it loses its luster, problems may be present. Redness of the eardrum or the ear canal is one of the first signs for which a doctor looks. However, redness of the eardrum is not a reliable basis for diagnosing a mid-dle ear infection.[11] Redness can occur because of allergy, high fever, inflammation or infection. Crying, which is typical of a sick child undergoing a middle ear exam, can lead to a temporary engorge-ment of the blood vessels in the ear canal and also can give a bright red appearance to the eardrum. This should not be mistaken for an ear infection.

A variation of the otoscope is the pneumatic otoscope. This device is an otoscope that has been modified by attaching a tube that connects to a small bulb. In an examination, the doctor places the speculum in the ear as usual. A tight seal of the speculum against the ear canal is needed so that no air escapes. The doctor then pumps air into the external ear chamber using the bulb. Pumping air into this sealed chamber causes the normal eardrum to be forced away from the doctor. When the air pressure is released, the eardrum returns to its normal position. If the middle ear is full of fluid or pus, the eardrum moves very little or not at all. When done properly, pneumatic otoscopy is a very useful way to find out if there is fluid in the middle ear.

Tympanometry is another method used to examine for middle ear effusion or fluid. Like the pneumatic otoscope, the tympanometer uses air pumped into the ear canal to assess movement of the eardrum. The major difference is that as air is drawn out of the ear canal, a sonic signal is bounced off the eardrum. As the air is gradually released, the response of the eardrum is monitored electronically and plotted on a graph—called a tympanogram. You may have heard your doctor refer to a "flat" tympanogram, meaning that the response of the eardrum to tympanometry did not produce the typical spiked curve. This suggests there is middle ear fluid.

Tympanometry is considered by many to be the most reliable means to determine the presence of middle ear fluid. Otoscopy alone is considered by many doctors to be less reliable than tympanometry alone. Perhaps the most thorough form of assessment of the middle ear is a combination of tympanometry with visual inspection using the otoscope. Because tympanometry equipment has become relatively inexpensive many clinics now use it in the evaluation of patients with middle ear complaints. One caveat is in order, however. A poor seal of the ear canal can lead to a "flat" tympanogram suggesting middle ear fluid is present when it is not. If you get a reading of a flat tympanogram, it may help to repeat it just to be sure.

Reflectometry is an accurate and simple method that relies on soundwaves to detect fluid in the middle ear.

All of these methods are used to varying degrees.

Terminology

There are a number of technical terms used throughout this book, and by your doctor, to describe earaches. Some of these may sound confusing. The medical term for problems of the middle ear is **otitis media**, derived from the Latin, oto- meaning ear, and -itis meaning inflammation. The term media means middle. Thus, otitis media technically means middle ear inflammation—not infection.

Other commonly used terms to describe illness involving the middle ear include:

Chronic and Acute: Refer to duration.
Chronic conditions are those that are recurrent and of long-standing duration. Acute conditions are usually associated with severe symptoms and are of short duration. A child can have chronic otitis media and still suffer from acute episodes.

Serous, Mucoid, and Purulent: Refer to the type of fluid present. Serous fluid is thin and watery, and usually does not contain harmful bacteria. This type of fluid is very common. Mucoid fluid is thick, sticky, and mucus-like. Purulent (also called suppurative) refers to the presence of fluid that contains many white blood cells— what we typically call pus. This is the type that usually contains harmful bacteria.

Effusion: Refers to the escape of fluid into the middle ear.

Doctors combine the above terms to describe the part involved, the specific region, whether it contains fluid, the type of fluid, and the duration of the problem. For instance, a diagnosis of chronic serous otitis media with effusion implies that there is fluid drainage into the middle ear that is recurring and of long-standing duration.

Throughout this book, I will use the terms earache, otitis media, and ear infection interchangeably. I continue to use the term ear infection out of familiarity to the reader. This term is often used inappropriately since not all earaches result from bacterial infection. As we'll see in chapter 5, the middle ear fluid in a high percentage of cases of otitis media contains either *no* bacteria, or *normal* bacteria. In only a small percentage of cases does it contain viruses. Therefore, recognize that not all "ear infections" are actually infections.

Who's at Risk

There are numerous factors that can put your child a increased risk to developing middle ear infection or inflammation. You may be able to reduce your child's chances of developing ear infections by addressing those risk factors that apply to her. Recognize that doctors disagree on the importance of some risk factors.

Season. The incidence of earaches is clearly highest in the winter, with the frequency decreasing in both spring and fall, and declining further in the summer. In northern climates, ear problems become more frequent beginning in September and begin to subside by April.[12]

Cow's Milk Consumption. Early consumption of cow's milk appears to predispose a child to early otitis media. Cow's milk consumption is one of the most significant contributors to middle ear problems in children.[13]

Feeding Position. In one study of more than 2,500 children, the practice of giving a child a bottle in bed was the most important factor associated with persistent fluid in the middle ear.[14] This is, in part, due to the horizontal position of the eustachian tube, and the ease with which fluid backs up into the tube. (See figure 1-b.)

Smoking. Children living in homes where one or more adult smokes develop otitis media at a much higher rate than children living in homes without smokers.[15]

Fetal Alcohol Exposure. A child whose mother has consumed alcohol during gestation is at high risk to developing fetal alcohol syndrome. Otitis media occurs in as many as 93 percent of children with fetal alcohol syndrome.[16]

Genetics. Nearly 60 percent of all children with Down syndrome suffer from otitis media.[17] (See chapter 6.)

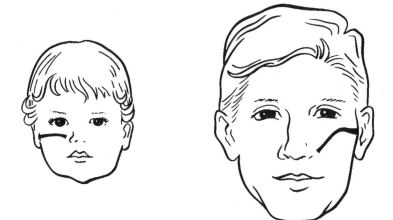

Figure 1-b
Comparison of the Infant and Adult Eustachian Tube

Day Care. Children spending time in day care settings have twice the chance of developing otitis media as children minded at home, and are at increased risk to developing illnesses of all types.[18]

Allergy. Many studies show that children with a personal or family history of allergy are more likely to develop otitis media than non-allergic children.[19]

Nutritional Status. Children with deficiency of certain vitamins, minerals, and fatty acids are at a risk to developing middle ear problems.[20]

Respiratory Problems. Nearly 50 percent of all cases of otitis media are preceded by an upper respiratory problem of some type (bronchial congestion, nasal congestion, asthma, colds, etc.).[21]

Injury. Children suffering trauma at birth such as that due to forceps, vacuum extraction, or prolonged and difficult labor are at risk to developing otitis media. Included in this category are children who have taken falls and suffered minor injury to the head and neck.[22]

Early Introduction of Solids. Middle ear problems often begin shortly after a baby begins to eat solid foods. The earlier solids are introduced, the greater the likelihood of developing otitis media.

Early Episodes of Otitis Media. Children who experience their first episode of otitis media in the first year of life are more likely to suffer from multiple recurrences of middle ear problems and persistent fluid.[23]

Low Socioeconomic Status. Children living in low socioeconomic conditions are at increased risk to those learning problems and developmental delays that are reported to occur in some children with recurrent otitis media.[24]

Current Medical Treatment

The medical treatment of otitis media involves a two-tiered approach consisting of drugs and surgery. Among the drugs used are antibiotics, antihistamines, and decongestants. Anti-inflammatory agents are often used to manage fever and pain. The surgical methods include tonsillectomy, adenoidectomy, myringotomy, and tympanostomy. When to use each of these approaches and for what length of time depends largely upon the individual doctor. As one prominent researcher states, "Recommendations regarding the management of secretory otitis media must be based to a considerable extent on opinion."[25] Recognize that new research, much of which has been reviewed in the treatment guidelines published by the United States Department of Health and Human Services, Agency for Health Care Policy Research, suggests that many common treatments are not effective. In several cases, they state that previously accepted treatments are "... not recommended." If one includes the European research, we are left with the understanding that all of the methods used to treat middle ear problems in children have been called into question. While some have selected value in some children, many have never been conclusively shown to be safe or effective.[26]

Thus, parents and doctors should weigh the evidence carefully, consider their options thoughtfully, and choose a course of action that is tailored to the individual child. The treatments and a brief note about each are listed below.

Antibiotics

According to estimates by the Centers for Disease Control, roughly 99 percent of children with otitis media receive antibiotics. This is in sharp contrast to European countries where antibiotic use is dramatically lower. Questions of antibiotic-resistant bacteria, side-effects of antibiotic drugs, and lack of effectiveness have caused physicians to take a halting look at the use of these drugs.

In chapter 2, we explore the benefits, risks, and effectiveness of antibiotics. The emerging picture is startling given the extent to which antibiotics are used on young children.

Cortisone

Cortisone is not widely used in otitis media. However, because many earaches are due to inflammation rather than infection, cortisone continues to be investigated as a therapeutic tool. Cortisone is used to treat the inflammatory aspects of otitis media. It works by interfering with the manufacture of a group of compounds known as inflammatory prostaglandins. (See chapter 5.)

Some reports have shown an increase in middle ear problems when cortisone is used. According to the treatment guidelines set forth by the Agency for Health Care Policy and Research, "Steroid medications are not recommended for treatment of otitis media with effusion in a child of any age." Only in the U.S. is the use of steroids even advocated for middle ear problems.[27]

Anti-Inflammatory Agents (Aspirin, Tylenol)

Drugs such as aspirin and acetaminophen (found in Tylenol) are not used as a principal therapy in otitis media, but are used freely to manage some of the symptoms and discomfort associated with earache including aches, pains, and fever. However, use of these drugs may actually prolong illness and lead to more inflammation. According to Dr. T.T.K. Jung, anti-inflammatory drugs may cause a case of secretory otitis media to degenerate into a case of mucoid otitis media[28] (one that is more resistant to treatment). In other words, if you use aspirin to make your child more comfortable during an ear infection, there is a chance that the middle ear will get worse and take longer to heal. (See chapter 5.)

This evidence is supported by recent findings reported in the *Journal of Pediatrics,* where acetaminophen (Tylenol) was shown to prolong the course of chicken pox. Many doctors now believe that acetaminophen also may prolong the course of other childhood infections, and that pain and fever reducers such as this should be used sparingly.[29]

Doctors have for some time recommended against giving aspirin to small children during an infection, because of the possibility that aspirin may trigger the development of Reye's syndrome. Reye's syndrome is an often-fatal inflammation of the brain.

Antihistamines/Decongestants

Theoretically, antihistamines should have value in the treatment of otitis media, at least in cases that are believed to be related to allergy. (Antihistamines block the release of histamine, and histamine release by white blood cells is part of the allergic response.) It is also logical that decongestants might work because they dry up the mucous membranes. However, some studies have shown that these drugs are of limited value in treating otitis media. The issue seems to have been settled by a careful analysis of existing studies done by a panel convened in 1994 by the U.S. department of Health and Human Services. The guidelines panel concluded that antihistamines and decongestants failed to have a statistically significant effect in improving otitis media with effusion, or chronic middle ear problems. They stated that "... antihistamines and decongestants are not recommended for otitis media with effusion."[30]

Tympanostomy

Tympanostomy refers to the placement of tubes in the eardrum. While this procedure is the most common surgery performed on children, many doctors believe it's used too frequently. Recent clinical trials have reported conflicting results regarding the effectiveness of tympanostomy. This is discussed in detail in chapter 3.

Tonsillectomy

The removal of tonsils was once the preferred surgical method of treating otitis media, but has now been replaced by tympanostomy. Swollen tonsils can obstruct the eustachian tube, thereby preventing the middle ear from draining properly. Doctors believe that by removing the tonsils, the eustachian tube opening becomes unblocked, leading to a reduction in middle ear fluid. However, many studies show that tonsillectomy does not affect the long-term course of otitis media.

The tonsils are essential lymphoid structures that play an important role in protecting the ear, nose, and throat area from bacteria and viruses that may gain entrance through the nose or mouth. Thus, removal of tonsils may increase susceptibility to infections of the ear, nose, and throat. The view of tonsillectomy has changed dramatically in recent years. Though some doctors still perform this surgery, it is not recommended as a treatment for otitis media. The AHCPR guidelines state that "Tonsillectomy should not be performed, either alone or with adenoidectomy, for the treatment of otitis media with effusion in a child of any age."[31,32]

Adenoidectomy

The adenoids are lymphoid structures located near the tonsils and the opening of the eustachian tube. Removal of adenoids is performed to "unblock" the eustachian tube opening. A number of studies show that this procedure has no effect on middle ear fluid or infection, and has little effect on the long-term course of otitis media. This is especially true in children with a history of allergy.[33,34,35,36]

According to the AHCPR guidelines, adenoidectomy is not recommended in children under three when there is no specific adenoid disease. In older children, effectiveness has not been proven.[37] (See chapter 3.)

Myringotomy

Myringotomy is performed by making an incision in the eardrum. The purpose is to relieve pressure within the middle ear cavity and allow fluid to escape. Sometimes myringotomy is performed alone. It is also the first step taken before the insertion of tubes. As with other surgical procedures in otitis media, it has not been conclusively shown to be effective. Members of a medical consensus conference recently concluded that "no convincing data from clinical trials have been reported to support the value of myringotomy with or without antimicrobial therapy for acute otitis media." Two studies at the University of Pittsburgh led to the conclusion that myringotomy is an unnecessary surgical procedure.[38] The only advantage of myringotomy appears to be pain relief, and this occurs in only a small percentage of children.[39]

One problem associated with myringotomy is that the incision in the eardrum often heals quickly. If the underlying disease has not been effectively treated, middle ear effusion quickly returns.[40]

In roughly one-fifth of all ear infections, the eardrum ruptures without intervention. Myringotomy is often used to prevent spontaneous rupture of the eardrum in the belief that an incision in the eardrum heals more efficiently than a rupture. However, ruptures usually heal completely within two weeks. Some doctors feel ruptures are not generally a cause for concern.[41]

Watchful Waiting

Doctors in Europe commonly use a policy of "watchful waiting" in children with otitis media. This means they do not rush to antibiotic or surgical treatment, but recommend pain relievers and allow the child to heal on her own. They also periodically monitor the child's condition as well as hearing levels. Only recently have the U.S. guidelines advocated watchful waiting as a sensible approach. There are estimates that 60 to 90 percent of cases of earache will heal without specific treatment.[42]

Complications of Otitis Media

Temporary and permanent injury to structures within the middle ear chamber are among the possible complications of otitis media. These include: scarring of the eardrum; thickening of the eardrum; permanent rupture of the eardrum; growth of polyps, granules, or cholesteatoma (the formation of a cyst-like mass filled with cholesterol and cells); tympanosclerosis (see chapter 3); and hearing loss. These complications can occur with or without treatment, although adequate treatment usually reduces the likelihood of complications. There is evidence (discussed in chapter 3) that certain treatments may even encourage the development of some of the above complications.

One of the most common complications of otitis media is mastoiditis. The mastoid is part of the temporal bone and is located just behind the ear. Within the temporal bone reside all of the structures of the middle ear. When infection or inflammation of the middle ear becomes severe, it can spread into what are called the mastoid air cells. The signs of mastoiditis include:[43]

- Thick pus discharging from the middle ear.
- Ear pushed out with sagging of the ear canal.
- Redness over the mastoid process.
- Mastoid tenderness.
- Fever, headache.
- X-ray evidence of breakdown of the mastoid's cellular partitions.

These symptoms are not always present. According to Dr. C.R. Pfaltz, antibiotics have changed the course of mastoiditis. Many of the specific signs that used to be associated with mastoiditis are often masked by the use of antibiotics.[44]

Mastoiditis can be followed by other complications. The most common among these is meningitis, which results when an infection has spread from the mastoid to the covering of the brain known as the meninges. Meningitis is a serious illness that requires the immediate attention of a physician and antibiotic treatment. Symptoms of meningitis include:

- Headache.
- Neck stiffness.
- Lethargy.
- Sleepiness.

- Loss of appetite.
- Vomiting.
- Fever.
- Chills.

Incidentally, the incidence of meningitis due to *Haemophilus influenzae* (a common ear-infecting bacteria) has risen by several hundred percent in some parts of the country, in spite of the widespread use of antibiotics to treat otitis media.[45]

Other complications of otitis media include: brain abscess, sigmoid sinus thrombosis, labyrinthitis. In a review of the complications of otitis media, Dr. Jack Froom states, ". . . fortunately [these complications] are very infrequent." When these complications occur, they usually require antibiotic intervention.[46]

Treatment of Otitis Media in Countries Other than the United States

Other countries with advanced health care systems have well-established treatment guidelines. In general, these countries use a far less aggressive approach to the treatment of otitis media. They consider drugs and surgery to be the last, rather than first resort.

For parents struggling with the dilemma of recurrent otitis media in their child, it should give some comfort to know that millions of children around the world are treated without drugs and surgery and, further, that this practice has not resulted in an epidemic of the complications once predicted. (This based on evidence to be shared later.) A few brief quotes from selected European guidelines are given below.

"Watchful waiting [no drugs] is the approach of choice for all children older than one year. . . . Analgesics [pain relievers] are the preferred symptomatic treatment at this moment."[47]

In two recent reports from the United Kingdom it is recognized that, "... unless children with OME are assessed symptomatically and repeatedly, a considerable proportion will undergo unwarranted surgery, with little or no resulting benefit.... There is no consistent evidence from randomized clinical trials that medical therapy including nasal decongestants, mucolytic agents, or antibiotics significantly affects the natural rate of resolution."[48]

In a report in the *British Medical Journal* entitled "Less Surgery for Glue Ear Says Bulletin," the panel states, "Because most children will recover spontaneously from glue ear [chronic middle ear effusion], a period of watchful waiting with a range of high quality hearing tests at the beginning and end is recommended."[49]

The Swedish Medical Research Council consensus statement on otitis media does not advocate drug therapy at all. It states, "Secretory otitis media heals spontaneously in most cases. The need for therapy should be individually assessed in children where a hearing impairment influences communications, speech, and language development, or interaction with their environment."[50]

According to Dr. Erdem Cantekin, the medical literature of other countries such as Denmark, Norway, and Switzerland could also be cited for advocating a similar approach: no antibiotics; surgery reserved for cases of prolonged hearing impairment.[51]

In the following chapters, we will explore antibiotics and surgery, and share some of the evidence that compels us to be cautious about their use. We will then embark on a discussion that will give new insight into the causes of middle ear problems and to the many possible solutions that exist.

Chapter 2

Antibiotics:
Sensible Use or Abuse?

*It is no accident that the most allergic generation in history
has been raised on antibiotics. Several times a week I see a
new patient whose allergies appeared or became much worse
after a course of antibiotics.*[1]

Leo Galland, M.D.

The editor of the journal *Clinical Otolaryngology* once wrote that
"... otitis media is a self-limiting disease, which is not affected by
any of the current methods of treatment."[2] There are two important considerations in his statement. First, self-limiting means that
a condition will usually run its course and improve over time. If
otitis media is indeed self-limiting, are doctors justified in using
the aggressive forms of antibiotic treatment we're accustomed to
seeing? Second, if otitis media is not affected by current methods
of treatment, does it not cast further doubt on the need for such
extensive antibiotic use on children with otitis media?

To put this in perspective, consider the history of antibiotic use.
At the time antibiotics were discovered, there were a number of
serious infectious diseases that claimed the lives of hundreds of
thousands of people. Infections from contagion and trauma were
rendered seemingly impotent by the long-awaited miracle drugs
called antibiotics. With their new-found arsenal, doctors slowly
began to expand the use of antibiotics to include the treatment of
bacterial diseases that were not life-threatening. Eventually anti-

biotics crept into use for almost any condition in which bacteria were thought to be involved. This included relatively minor conditions such as otitis media.

We then saw the evolution (one might arguably call it regression) to prophylactic, or preventive antibiotic prescribing. In cases that were often of viral origin, children were given antibiotics to "prevent a secondary bacterial infection."

Prior to the antibiotic era, roughly 80 percent of all ear infections resolved spontaneously.[3] Today, nearly 9 out of 10 children diagnosed with middle ear infection will receive an antibiotic for their condition. Perhaps this antibiotic use is justified. Perhaps it's not.

In the management of any illness, doctors must always consider the so-called risk/benefit ratio. If a child suffers from middle ear infection, does he face a greater risk from the disease or the antibiotic? For decades, doctors were unquestioning in their belief that the risks of otitis media far outweighed the risk of antibiotics. Antibiotics were thought to be benevolent substances that imparted only good to the patient. However, we now know that antibiotics are a double-edged sword.

In spite of this knowledge, antibiotics are prescribed to children with more zeal today than ever before. From 1977 to 1986, antibiotic prescriptions to children under age 10 increased an alarming 51 percent, while the number of children in this age group grew by only 9 percent. In contrast, antibiotic prescriptions to the general population declined substantially during this time.[4]

According to Wendy Nelson, of the FDA's epidemiology and surveillance office, in 1977, 26 percent of all antibiotics were prescribed for otitis media. By 1986, the diagnosis of otitis media accounted for 42 percent of all antibiotics prescribed to pediatric outpatients. Antibiotic prescriptions to children under three showed the most dramatic increase.[5]

Amoxicillin, the most frequently prescribed drug for otitis media, now has the distinction of being the most frequently prescribed antibiotic of all—accounting for 21 percent of antibiotics used in 1986. A report published in Medical World News (1987) showed that, in the pediatric population, broad-spectrum penicillins and sulfa-containing drugs accounted for roughly 65 percent of all antibiotics prescribed in 1986.[6]

These figures provide reason for concern because of the potential hazards associated with the liberal use of antibacterial drugs. Among the most commonly cited problems with antibiotic use are:

- Antibiotic use can lead to the development of antibiotic-resistant bacteria.

- Antibiotics are associated with many adverse physical effects.

- There is conflicting information regarding whether antibiotics are effective for the majority of children with otitis media.

- There is uncertainty over the value of prophylactic (preventive) antibiotics.

- We don't fully understand the impact of the additional antibiotics children are exposed to through the food supply.

Parents need to take these issues seriously because not all doctors do.

Antibiotic-Resistant Bacteria

Indiscriminate use of antibiotics is leading us to one of the most frightening eras in recent memory. That is, the return of infectious diseases for which there is no cure. Two decades following the introduction of antibiotics, doctors began to observe an alarming trend. Infectious diseases that were once treatable no longer responded to antibiotics. Those that did respond often required five to ten times the amount of the drug that used to be effective. The reason— bacteria were developing resistance to the drugs.

In response to this surge in antibiotic-resistant bacteria, pharmaceutical researchers developed a new array of antibiotics against which the bacteria had no resistance. Over time, bacteria developed resistance to the new drugs as well. According to Dr. Marc Lappé in

When Antibiotics Fail, by 1960 roughly 80 percent of the tested *staphylococcal* organisms showed resistance to penicillin, tetracycline, and chloramphenicol. Today, penicillin can kill only 10 percent of the varieties of *Staphylococcus aureus* that it used to dispose of easily.[7]

Gonorrhea was once easily cured with moderate doses of penicillin. Today, however, it takes several substantial doses of penicillin to cure the disease. More frightening is the number of resistance strains of gonorrhea that have popped up around the world that do not respond to penicillin at all.

Regarding the antibiotic resistance crisis, Dr. Alexander Tomasz of Rockefeller University warned that scientists expect "nothing short of a medical disaster." Dr. Bill Jarvis, of the Centers for Disease Control and Prevention stated that the antibiotic resistance crisis "... is probably the No. 1 public health issue."

The earliest association with antibiotic resistance and otitis media appeared in a paper entitled " The Increasing Incidence of Ampicillin-Resistant Haemophilus Influenzae: a Cause of Otitis Media." *Haemophilus influenzae* is one of the most commonly found bacteria in infected middle ear fluid. In this report, Dr. R. Schwartz and his colleagues observed that in 1975, only one ampicillin-resistant strain of *H. influenzae* was isolated from the middle ear fluid of children in their study. By 1976, 18 percent of all *H. influenzae* had become resistant to ampicillin. Midway through 1977, the percentage of ampicillin-resistant *H. influenzae* had grown to 35 percent — an almost 35 percent increase in just two years.[8]

The trend in bacterial development of antibiotic resistance is not unlike the increasing resistance of agricultural pests to pesticides. In 1938, scientists knew of just seven insect and mite species that had acquired resistance to pesticides. by 1984, that figure had climbed to 447 and included most of the world's major pests. In response to heavier pesticide use and a wider variety of pesticides, pests have evolved sophisticated mechanisms for resisting the action of chemicals designed to kill them.[9] Pesticides also kill the pests' natural enemies, much like antibiotics kill the natural enemies of harmful bacteria in the body.

Antibiotic resistance often develops in bacteria when they are repeatedly exposed to an antibiotic. Children who have received repeated courses of ampicillin, or other antibiotics in the penicillin group, harbor more antibiotic-resistant *Haemophilus influenzae* than those with little or no exposure to these drugs. Also, ampicillin-resistant strains of *H. influenzae* are reported more often in children with otitis media that is relapsing, recurrent, or chronic than in children with an initial infection.[10]

In a study of children who had been previously treated with ampicillin, 46 percent of those with *H. influenzae* in their middle ear had become resistant to ampicillin, and 100 percent with *M. catarrhalis* were resistant.[11]

Not only do antibiotic-resistant bacteria pass the tools for resistance among their species, but from one species to another. This allows ampicillin-resistant *H. influenzae*, for example, to pass the gene for resistance (called an R-plasmid) to other *H. influenzae*, to common strep bacteria in the throat, to normal intestinal bacteria, or to any number of other organisms as well.

Antibiotic-resistant bacteria in the environment or the intestine also can pass on their tolls for resistance. Consider the common intestinal bacteria *E. coli*. According the Dr. H. G. Welch, a specialist in the study of antibiotic resistance, *E. coli* is one of the most frequently resistant bacteria to both ampicillin and amoxicillin. This bacteria has the ability to pass the genes for resistance to either *H. influenzae* or *Streptococcus pneumoniae*—two common ear-infecting bacteria.

In *Postgraduate Medicine,* Dr. Welch comments that "... antibiotic use, while contributing to the immediate demise of bacteria, serves to 'educate' microbes by establishing selective pressure that favors the 'smarter' bacteria, i.e., those that can resist the antibiotic."[12] Antibiotics such as ampicillin destroy susceptible *H. influenzae* in the middle ear, but the handful that remain are resistant to the drug. They reproduce and before long there is a large colony of resistant bacteria.

The consequences of antibiotic resistance can be serious. In one Minnesota hospital, patients who harbored antibiotic-resistant staph bacteria required hospital stays 43 days longer than those with non-resistant staph. Those with resistant staph infections also had a higher mortality rate.[13] As this study shows, antibiotic resistance can lead to diseases that are not responsive to any form of therapy.

Haemophilus influenzae is a sobering example. This bacteria is not only associated with middle ear infection, but with meningitis and epiglottitis as well. Meningitis is a serious inflammation of the brain that must be treated with antibiotics. Epiglottitis is a serious and life-threatening disease that occurs when *H. influenzae* type b causes the epiglottis to swell, which closes off the airway resulting in suffocation. (The epiglottis is a cartilaginous flap that prevents food and water from entering the lungs during swallowing.) It too must be treated vigorously and rapidly with antibiotics. However, if the bacteria are resistant to the antibiotic being used, the disease will not respond to treatment. Herein lies the most serious dilemma of antibiotic overuse. When life-threatening illness occurs, will the bacteria succumb to our drugs?

Adverse Physical Effects of Antibiotics

When antibiotics are used, there is often a trade-off between benefits and adverse physical effects. Sometimes the need for the antibiotic outweighs the risk of these physical effects, and the use of the drug is justified. When antibiotics are used excessively, the physical harm often offsets the benefits of the drug. Listed below are some adverse effects associated with antibiotics.

Destruction of Helpful Intestinal Bacteria

The common intestinal bacteria *Lactobacillus acidophilus* and *Bifidobacterium bifidus* are essential to proper digestive function, immune function, and synthesis of certain vitamins.[14] In addition, they protect us from infections of the intestinal tract. Most antibiotics are undiscriminating with regard to intestinal bacteria. When antibiotics are used, *L. acidophilus* and *B. bifidus* are among the first to be killed. (The important functions of these bacteria are discussed in chapter 6.) Many physicians have not given this issue serious consideration. However, it is not for lack of evidence. An article in the *Journal of Chemotherapy* reviewed the adverse intestinal effects of dozens of commonly used antibiotics. The authors state, "The most common and significant cause of disturbance in the normal intestinal microflora is the administration of antimicrobial agents.... In most cases, the influence is not beneficial to the patient."[15]

Increased Susceptibility to Intestinal Infection

Because of the adverse effect on *L. acidophilus, B. bifidus,* and the local immune system, antibiotics can cause children to be more susceptible to parasitic infection. For instance, infection by the parasite *Giardia lamblia* is made easier following the administration of antibiotics. *G. lamblia* is one of the most common waterborne parasites in the United States, affecting an estimated 18 million people.[16] *Giardia* is also listed among the top ten most common infectious agents found in day care centers.[17] In addition to the intestinal problems created, parasitic infection causes immune suppression, which often leads to increased susceptibility to subsequent bacterial infection.[18]

Antibiotic use also can result in an overgrowth of the bacterium *Clostridium dificile* in the colon. This has been linked with the development of a painful inflammatory condition known as pseudomembranous colitis.[19]

A yeast organism that normally lives in the intestinal tract—and is kept in check by *L. acidophilus* and *B. bifidus*—overgrows following excessive antibiotic use. This yeast, called *Candida albicans,* is responsible for the development of food allergy, environmental sensitivity, and recurring infections.[20] *Candida albicans* also adds to intestinal problems by stimulating the growth of *Giardia lamblia.*[21]

The ability of antibiotics to increase susceptibility to intestinal parasites is a serious matter because parasitic infection of children in the United States is a growing problem. In one study of 321 children from Houston, Texas, 49.5 percent tested positive for intestinal parasites. The rate of infection is high in Houston in part because of its proximity to Mexico. However, the rate of parasitic infection of children in the general population is increasing nationwide. It is especially high in the Southwestern United States.[22]

Intestinal Inflammation, Leaky Gut, and Food Allergy

Among other things, the intestinal lining serves two important functions. It allows absorption of nutrients and prevents absorption of unwanted substances. When nutrients are poorly absorbed it is referred to as malabsorption. When unwanted substances are allowed to pass across the gut wall it is called **leaky gut,** or increased intestinal permeability. Excessive antibiotic exposure may indirectly disrupt the barrier and transport functions of the gut, which may contribute to inflammatory changes and leaky gut syndrome.

Increased intestinal permeability appears to be a critical factor in some people with food allergy. In a recent study it was shown that people with food allergy had increased intestinal permeability and that when offending foods were introduced the permeability (leakiness) further worsened. During periods of fasting or allergen avoidance, altered permeability improved.

Many children who experience chronic middle ear effusion do so because of food allergy. (See Chapter 5.) Food allergy may exist, in some children, because of increased intestinal permeability. Increased intestinal permeability may exist, in part, because of antibiotic overuse.

If this pattern exists in a child, additional antibiotic use may further disrupt intestinal balance, which may aggravate the leaky gut syndrome. This may, in turn, increase reactivity to foods, which may contribute to continued middle ear effusion. It may be one reason why children with recurrent earaches who take repeated courses of antibiotics either do not improve or get worse—the antibiotic may aggravate the underlying syndrome.[23,24]

The presence of leaky gut can be determined using a test that measures the uptake of the substances lactulose and mannitol. Great Smokies Diagnostic Laboratory in Asheville, North Carolina currently offers such a test, which must be ordered by your doctor. If it is established that leaky gut syndrome exists, nutritional protocols can be tailored to restore intestinal integrity.

Inhibition of Immunity

Antibiotics can inhibit the ability of white blood cells (called neutrophils) to protect against the overgrowth of *Candida albicans*.[25] Once an infestation of *Candida albicans* gets out of control, multiple health problems typically follow. Children who have had repeated doses of antibiotics for recurrent otitis media, but have failed to improve, often suffer from a secondary problem caused by *Candida albicans*. Under these circumstances, further antibiotic use severely aggravates the situation. Usually such children will not improve until antibiotics are discontinued and the yeast problems are addressed.

Some antibiotics prevent neutrophil chemotaxis.[26] When-ever an infectious agent is present in the body, chemical signals are sent out that tell the white blood cells where to go, a process called chemotaxis.

When white blood cells do get to the site of infection, they often release peroxides (such as hydrogen peroxide) that essentially "bleach" the bacteria to death. Some antibiotics reduce the ability of white blood cells to destroy bacteria in this way.[27]

Antibiotics can also depress natural killer cell activity and reduce the production of antibodies.[28] The depressed antibody production is important since antibodies are produced in response to a bacteria as a means of signaling the body to kill it. Antibodies also provide a "memory" of invading bacteria. With this memory in place, the likelihood of succumbing to future infection by that bacteria is sharply reduced. When the memory is not sufficient, reinfection is more likely. Some antibiotics delay the antibody response. Frequently, the delay may last for up to 20 days after the antibiotic has been discontinued.[29]

In an article published in The American Journal of Medicine in 1982, Drs. William Hauser and Jack Remington of Stanford University School of Medicine reported on the ability of some antibiotics to alter the immune response. Tetracycline was shown to inhibit the ability of white cells to engulf and destroy bacteria (phagocytosis) and to delay the ability of white cells to move to the site of infection. Sulfonamides inhibited the microbiocidal activity of white cells. Trimethoprim-sulfamethoxazole inhibited antibody production. Similar action of numerous antibiotics was reported.

Such studies do not suggest that antibiotics should never be used, but they are strong evidence that doctors must seriously consider the risks and benefits when prescribing.[30]

Reduced Absorption of Nutrients

There is some evidence that certain antibiotics reduce the absorption of nutrients such as vitamin K, vitamin B12, folic acid, calcium, and magnesium.[31] These effects may be minimal in children who are healthy or when antibiotic therapy is short-term. However, children who receive repeated doses of antibiotics or who suffer intestinal symptoms (such as diarrhea) from antibiotic therapy may experience losses of nutrients that can impair their ability to fight infection. The adverse affects of antibiotics on nutrients is likely to be greatest when: 1) broad-spectrum antibiotics are used, 2) repeated courses of antibiotics are used, 3) prophylactic or preventive antibiotics are used, and 4) the child has a history of malabsorption or intestinal disease.

Antibiotics and Developmental Delays

Some professionals who work with children suffering from developmental delays have speculated that long-term antibiotic use (or short-term use of some very powerful antibiotics) may actually contribute to neurologic impairment and developmental delay. Kelly Dorfman, M.S. and Patricia Lemer, M.ed., co-founders of the Developmental Delay Registry in Chevy Chase, Maryland, are among those who have observed the developmental decline of some children following antibiotic therapy.

Their observation, guided by consultation with an international medical advisory board, led them to conduct a national pilot survey aimed at determining if the subject warranted further research. It should be noted that determining an association between a broad class of drugs and non-specific developmental delays is a very challenging and difficult research effort with many potential pitfalls. However, the stakes are so potentially high that the question needs to be asked.

The pilot survey of 696 children (449 delayed, 247 normally

developing) led to the following conclusion: "The strong correlation between these three factors —maternal health, recurrent childhood ear infections, treatment with antibiotics —and developmental delays is impressive. Children on prophylactic antibiotics were 50 percent more likely to be in the developmentally delayed group. Although the DDR study does not provide a basis for a clear statement of a cause and effect relationship, further investigation is clearly warranted."[32]

Lending further credence to the hypothesis that antibiotics may contribute developmental delays in susceptible children is the preliminary data from a group working in collaboration with the University of Missouri School of Medicine. Drs. William Shaw and his colleagues at Children's Mercy Hospital in Kansas City, initially studied two autistic boys who had frequent ear infections and a long history of antibiotic use. Their autistic symptoms emerged around age two. Organic acid analysis of urine revealed several unusual products, which could not be accounted for by any human metabolic process. Shaw learned that these metabolites, which are neurotoxic, are products of yeast and fungal metabolism.[33]

The next step was to see if antifungal medication could lower the level of these organic acids in the urine of a larger group of autistic children. His groups' preliminary findings have shown that antifungal drugs (Nystatin® or Diflucan®) lower the level of these neurotoxic substances in the urine and improve some autistic symptoms. Parents of the children noted improvement such as decreased hyperactivity, better concentration, more eye contact, and other improvements.[34]

What is the potential significance of this work beyond autism? Antibiotics are known to produce disruption of intestinal organisms and allow for overgrowth of yeast and fungi. It is now known that some byproducts of intestinal bacterial metabolism can be absorbed into the bloodstream. The neurotoxins discovered in this group of autistic children are known fungal byproducts. The finding that potentially neurotoxic compounds could be lowered by antifungal drugs further suggests a fungal origin.

An important question must therefore be asked. Is it possible that a subcategory of susceptible children who are given antibiotics experience overgrowth of fungi in the gut, which then produce substances toxic to the nervous system? If so, it would explain why some children appear to experience developmental delay following antibiotic therapy.

That I have chosen to present such preliminary evidence before it is confirmed experimentally is likely to produce outrage among some physicians. While I agree there should be no rush to judgment, I think the findings are so potentially profound that they deserve debate in an open forum. We have no clear explanation for the rise in developmental delays in modern culture. While it is undoubtedly complex, I believe we must candidly discuss and investigate every possibility. Meanwhile, we must be certain that antibiotic therapy does not put any child at risk, especially in cases where the potential for gain is minimal.

Antibiotics and Otitis Media: Helpful for Most Children?

There is evidence suggesting that antibiotics are effective in managing some types of middle ear infections. Members of a 1984 conference entitled "Controversies in Antimicrobial Agents for Otitis Media," chaired by Charles D. Bluestone, M.D., suggest that antimicrobial therapy *is* indicated for acute otitis media. Sulfonamides have been shown to be somewhat effective in treating ear infections.[35] Amoxicillin was found, in one trial, to be more effective than placebo in treating acute otitis media.[36] Researchers in Canada, after a study of 142 children, concluded that penicillin and ampicillin were superior to symptomatic therapy.[37] However the percentage of children for whom antibiotics are useful may be low when compared with the number of children receiving antibiotics for otitis media. Supporting the latter contention are several studies conducted over the past two decades.

In many studies (as in daily practice), middle ear cultures are not performed to determine whether harmful bacteria exist.

Dr. S. A. Carlin and colleagues completed a study of of children who were culture-positive for common middle ear bacteria. Sensitivity tests were performed to determine sensitivity of the bacteria to six different antibiotics. Treating only the children who tested positive for bacteria, 86 percent showed improvement.[38] Unfortunately, the percentage of children for whom antibiotics are useful may be low when compared with the number of children receiving antibiotics for otitis media. Supporting the latter contention are several studies conducted over the past two decades.

In a recent study involving 3,660 children and physicians from nine countries, antibiotic-treated children recovered at a rate slightly slower than children not receiving antibiotics.[39] Dr. F. L. Van Buchem compared children treated with antibiotics, antibiotics and myringotomy or no treatment and found little difference between the groups with regard to pain, level of hearing, healing time, recurrence and fever.[40]

In another study, Dr. Van Buchem reported on a study of 4,860 children with acute otitis media treated with pain relievers and nose drops for four days (without antibiotics or myringotomy). *More than 90 percent of these children recovered in a few days with no need for further treatment.* Three percent of cases were severe and required antibiotic therapy. Van Buchem concluded "treatment of acute otitis media in children can be limited to nose drops and analgesics for the first three to four days. An antibiotic, preferably penicillin, can be given in the severe cases (still ill after three to four days with persistent high temperature or severe pain, or both) and to patients who do not clinically appear to be ill but still have discharge of the ear after two weeks."[41]

After studying nearly four thousand children, two Dutch physicians concluded that 88 percent of children with acute otitis media never need antibiotics. They showed that when antibiotic treatment was instituted within the first two days of illness the rate of recurrence was 2.9 percent greater than if antibiotic treatment was delayed up to eight days (1.3 percent) or not used.[42]

In an article in the *Journal of the American Medical Association*, researchers reported that children with chronic otitis media with effusion who received amoxicillin fared no better than those on placebo and, in fact, suffered two to six times greater recurrence than those on placebo. Similar findings were reported for Pediazole and cefaclor.[43]

Dr. John Bailar, the Scholar-in-Residence at the National Academy of Sciences' Institute of Medicine and editorial board member of the *New England Journal of Medicine,* reported on his analysis of the data regarding antibiotic treatment of otitis media. Commenting on the pattern of ineffectiveness he wrote, "This remarkable trend ... seems to demolish the conclusion that antibiotics improve the outcome [of otitis media]."[44]

A landmark article published in the *Journal of the American Medical Association* had this to say following an extensive analysis of the existing research on antibiotics and chronic middle ear problems: "Antibiotics appear to have beneficial but limited effect on recurrent otitis media and short term resolution of otitis media with effusion [OME]. Longer term benefit for OME has not been shown."

The authors go on to say that, "Because a major goal of treatment of OME is the prevention of language or developmental delays due to hearing deficits, the lack of long term effectiveness leads one to question the value of antibiotic treatment."[45]

In countries such as Sweden, antibiotic treatment of otitis media is viewed with great caution. According to Karin Prellner, M.D., of the Swedish Medical Research Council, it would be difficult to conduct a placebo-controlled trial using antibiotics in otitis media in Sweden because antibiotics are viewed as an ineffective and potentially harmful form of therapy. She suggested that doctors there would be faced with a serious ethical conflict if they were forced to give antibiotics for what they consider a benign disorder, i.e. otitis media without complications.[46]

Robert Ruben, M.D., President of the American Society for Pediatric Otolaryngology, gave an address in which he seriously questioned the value of antibiotics in otitis media on three grounds: lack of effectiveness, antibiotic-resistant bacteria, safety.

He stated, "It would appear that the widespread use of antibiotics for otitis media with effusion has added to the creation of antibiotic-resistant organisms throughout the world.... The creation of antibiotic-resistant organisms is now a medical and social problem that needs to be addressed and regulated."

Regarding effectiveness he states, "Overall, the effectiveness of antibiotics for all of the types of morbidities [illnesses] associated with otitis media with effusion is marginal or equal to that of placebo."

His harshest criticism was reserved for the side-effects of antibiotics when he remarked, "The sequelae [consequences] resultant from the use of antibiotics is substantial to both patient and society. Analysis of the data indicates that *antibiotics are an ineffective and dangerous form of care for otitis media with effusion.*" [Emphasis mine]

Length of Treatment

Doctors in the United States almost always prescribe antibiotics for 10 days when treating ear infections. No one is sure where this practice originated since there is no evidence in the medical literature that shows taking an antibiotic for this length of time is optimum. In fact, recent studies have shown that the results obtained following seven-day, five-day, three-day, or even two-day courses of antibiotics are comparable to those obtained when a 10-day course is prescribed. These shortened antibiotic regiments appear to carry no greater risk of complications from otitis media than the customary 10-day regimen.[47,48,49,50]

Preventing Complications

Among the most common arguments in favor of antibiotics is that they have reduced the rate of complications (such as mastoiditis and meningitis) encountered in otitis media. This is a reasonable assertion with which most doctors would agree. However, Dutch researcher F.L. Van Buchem, M.D., contends that "no conclusion can be drawn, from the published work, on the influence of antibiotics on the incidence of mastoiditis."[51] In spite of the great advances in antibiotic therapy, there has been an increase ranging from 3 to 400 percent (based on studies in the United States, Canada,

England, and Denmark) in the incidence of *Haemophilus influenzae* meningitis.[52]

When researchers compared Canada, where antibiotics are used aggressively to treat middle ear problems, with the Netherlands, where antibiotics are used much less frequently, they found virtually no difference in the occurrence of mastoiditis.[53,54] Perhaps most compelling is the result of a nationwide survey in Denmark, in which only 6 cases of mastoiditis were reported in 1994.[55] If the rationale for aggressive use of antibiotics is to prevent serious complications, yet comparisons show these complications do not occur to the degree once thought, the use of antibiotics becomes harder to justify. These data have caused doctors to seriously question their assumptions about the role and effectiveness of antibiotics under these circumstances.

Proper Use?

A final question surrounding the effectiveness of antibiotics is their proper use. The sobering comments of Dr. James Hughes of the Centers for Disease Control and Prevention truly bring the question of proper use into perspective. Hughes stated in 1995 that up to one half of the 110 million antibiotic prescriptions written each year may be "inappropriate" for the illness being treated.[56] In the journal Pediatrics, F. A. Disney, M.D., former president of the American Board of Pediatrics, discussed a telephone conference dealing with the choice and use of antibiotics. Disney remarked that he was "astonished" and "alarmed" at the methods that certified pediatricians in practice were using to select antibiotics. Most disconcerting were assertions that the antibiotic was commonly "picked at random or was selected by the doctor's preference for one drug or another chosen on the basis of available samples or side effects ..." One doctor stated that "if the child wasn't better by the end of a period of time, then all drugs were stopped and subsequently the child sometimes did recover." Dr. Disney suggested that in such cases "possibly the drugs were contributing to the child's illness."[57]

Accuracy of diagnosis is one final area of concern regarding the proper use of antibiotics. In order to recommend proper treatment, doctors must first make an accurate diagnosis of a child's condition. But doctors are not always certain of their diagnosis. Researchers from the International Primary Care Network found that doctors were certain of their diagnosis of otitis media in only 58 percent of children under twelve months.[58] This finding is of great concern since many children in which the diagnosis was uncertain undoubtedly received antibiotics. The low degree of diagnostic certainty is not necessarily the fault of doctors since children under twelve months are often difficult to examine. Yet, it adds to the dilemma of deciding when antibiotics are appropriate for children with otitis media.*

Preventive (Prophylactic) Antibiotics

Many doctors prescribe prophylactic antibiotics in the hope that an impending infection might be prevented. At first glance the practice seems rational. Marc Lappé, Ph.D., well-known pathologist and toxicologist, contends that prophylactic use of antibiotics comprises the "worst category of misuse."[59] He cites numerous studies that show 50 to 65 percent of prophylactically prescribed antibiotics are given inappropriately. According to Silverman and Lee in *Pills, Profit and Politics* (1974), "... the best thing that can be said about prophylactic antibiotics is that in most instances it is not clinically justifiable. It presents needless risks and unnecessary expense. At worst, it may be fatal for the patient."

Dr. Michael Persico and his associates found that prophlactic use of penicillin improved the clinical condition of recurrent acute otitis media. However, in the children who experienced a reduction in recurrent acute otitis media, there was no decrease in middle ear fluid. At all stages of follow-up, *there was no difference in middle ear appearance in those children* receiving prophylactic doses of penicillin when compared with those receiving a short course of

---

*Diagnostic certainty in children aged 13 to 30 months was 66 percent and 73 percent in those older than 30 months.

ampicillin.[60] According to Dr. M. Tos, "Antibiotic treatment does not promote the development of secretory otitis, but is probably unable to prevent it."[61]

A recent report showed that prophylactic doses of antibiotics* prescribed at night for several months reduced the frequency of recurrent episodes of otitis media. The beneficial effects appeared to be most significant for children under age two and children attending day care. This is encouraging. However, the degree to which middle ear effusion had declined after six months was nearly the same in the placebo group as in the antibiotic groups.[62]

There may be instances where prophylactic antibiotics are required. However, because of the numerous adverse effects associated with indiscriminate antibiotic use, children chosen for prophylactic antibiotics should be selected carefully. In the world of antibiotics and bacteria, a cavalier attitude toward prescribing is no longer acceptable.

Foodborne Antibiotics

The clinical use of antibiotics is unfortunately not our only source of exposure. Agricultural antibiotic sales account for nearly three-fourths of all antibiotics sold in the United States (243 million dollars annually by 1979).[63] The use of antibiotics has been reported on more than 90 percent of the beef, pork, and poultry in the U.S. Drug-resistant *Salmonella* are appearing in tainted beef, poultry, and milk at an increasing rate. The total incidence of disease transmission due to tainted food is unknown, since many mild intestinal symptoms go unreported, and tracing an outbreak to its source is costly and difficult.

According to Dr. Richard Novick, farm animals contribute between 99 and 99.9 percent of all the resistant coliform bacteria (especially *E. coli*) in the environment. In addition, he states that there are no barriers to the spread of genes for antibiotic resistance

---

*Amoxicillin and sulfamethoxazole with trimethoprim were compared with placebo in this study. (*American Journal of Diseases of Children*, 1989)

and that they pose "a substantial hazard to human health due to therapeutic compromise."[64]

In 1983, a midwestern outbreak of intestinal disease in 18 people was associated with an antibiotic-resistant form of *Salmonella newport* (resistant to ampicillin, carbenicillin, and tetracycline). The source of the infection was traced to hamburger in which chlortetracycline had been used for growth promotion. (The use of this antibiotic led to the development of antibiotic-resistant *S. newport*.) Twelve of the people had been taking penicillin-derived antibiotics in the 24- to 48-hour period before the onset of intestinal symptoms.

According to scientists at the State Health Departments in Minnesota and North Dakota, the patients had been infected before they took antibiotics. Their use of antibiotics, to which the *S. newport* was resistant, led to a reduction in the normal intestinal bacteria, resulting in more serious intestinal infection by *S. newport*.

Researchers in charge of this case conclude that "... anti-microbial-resistant organisms of animal origin cause serious human illness," and urge "... *far more prudent use of antimicrobials in both human beings* and animals"[emphasis mine].[65]

Antibiotics are used in animal feed to slightly enhance growth (by 5 to 6 percent). However, animals raised on antibiotic-treated feed serve as a reservoir of antibiotic-resistant bacteria. Over the years, scientists have observed a direct relationship between the number of resistant strains of bacteria appearing in animals and the use of antibiotics in animal feed. These antibiotic-resistant bacteria have appeared on meat and dairy products sold to consumers. When these products are consumed, the bacteria are passed into the intestinal tract of those who eat them. This is believed to be partially responsible for the increase in antibiotic-resistant bacteria in humans.

Antibiotic-resistant bacteria in our food is unfortunately not the only hazard associated with agricultural use of antibiotics. The drugs themselves are making their way into the food we feed our children.

A recent analysis done by the U.S. Congress' General Accounting Office has identified traces of 64 different antibiotics in cow's milk at levels "that raise health concerns." Antibiotic levels deemed safe by the Food and Drug Administration have been shown by scientists at Rutgers University to increase the rate at which antibiotic-resistant bacteria emerged by 600 to 2,700 percent.

Antibiotics used in animal husbandry also apparently cause the emergence of antibiotic-resistant microbes in family farmers, which can then be passed onto the community. In a study conducted by Tufts University, tetracycline given to chicks caused development of antibiotic-resistant strains of *E. coli.* after only a few days. During the next three months, the bacteria developed resistance to multiple antibiotics including ampicillin and streptomycin, even though these drugs had not been given. Over the next six months, the farmers harbored *E. coli* with the same resistance pattern. In a related study conducted in Germany, antibiotic resistance was passed from pigs, to farmers, and disturbingly, to members of the community who merely lived in the area.

Agricultural use of antibiotics results in drug residue and antibiotic-resistant bacteria in the food we eat. The effect of this type of low-grade, long-term exposure on children (or adults) is unclear. What is clear is that our use of antibiotics in medicine must take this additional exposure into account. You as a consumer of food should demand, through your purchasing power, that only antibiotic-free meat and milk be available. This can be done by purchasing food that is labeled organic or raised free of antibiotics. As consumers of health care, you should demand that your doctors give good rationale for their use of antibiotics on your child.

In Support of Antibiotics

This chapter is not written as a full-fledged assault on the use of antibiotics. The intent is to show parents and health care professionals the hazards of unbridled use of these drugs. No one desires to go back to the pre-antibiotic era when infectious diseases were rampant. But in our zeal to eradicate microbes at all costs, we may have unwittingly chosen the very course we have sought to avoid.

Antibiotics, when used wisely, are an extremely valuable weapon in the medical arsenal. When microorganisms threaten to over-whelm the defenses of a sick child, antibiotics should be used. When complications are present or imminent, antibiotics should be used. There are numerous circumstances under which prudent antibiotic use is to be considered in the management of otitis media and other diseases. Whether they are necessary for the treatment of your child can only be decided after careful consideration of the facts and con-sultation with your doctor.

If your doctor chooses to prescribe antibiotics, I believe it is essential that he or she also address dietary, nutritional, and other factors discussed in this book. When these factors are addressed, the effectiveness of any treatment should be enhanced, and the risk of recurrent infection reduced.

When illness arises in your family and the doctor recommends antibiotics, ask him or her the following questions.

1. Are you certain this is a bacterial infection? Could it be a virus?

2. Do you know the type of bacteria involved?

3. Have you determined to which antibiotic the bacteria is sensitive? Have you performed a sensitivity test?

4. What is the minimum amount of time that I must take the antibiotic in order for it to be effective?

5. Can we use an antibiotic with a narrow spectrum of action and still get the job done?

6. What are the expected side effects of taking this antibiotic?

7. Could we allow the immune system to do its work and use the antibiotic later? What are the consequences if I wait?

8. What are the likely consequences if I do not use antibiotics?

9. Are there alternatives to antibiotics? What other things might I do to optimize my child's immune response?

Your doctor may be reluctant or unable to answer these questions. However, if he or she gives you good reasons for proceeding with antibiotic therapy, you should follow this advice. If the doctor has not addressed the above questions or has not given you a satisfactory answer, you should be more cautious.

Chapter 3

Tubes: Effectiveness, Hazards, and Complications

*Incredibly, one of the side effects of this procedure, performed to cure recurrent otitis media, is **acute** otitis media.*[1]
Robert S. Mendelsohn, M.D.

Tympanostomy, or insertion of tubes in the eardrum, has rapidly emerged as the surgical method of choice in the treatment of childhood ear infections. Recent estimates show that tympanostomy is performed on more than one million children each year,[2] at an average cost of roughly 2,000 dollars per surgery. In many cases the surgery is performed on both ears, resulting in perhaps almost two million tubes annually. It is common for tubes to fall out prematurely, often within 4 to 7 months.[3,4] The recurrence of middle ear effusion following the rejection of tubes seems to occur in as high as 40 percent of all children. Of the children who prematurely reject their tubes, 33 to 75 percent require a second surgery to replace them.[5,6]

There is disagreement over whether tubes are effective, and if so, when their use should be considered. Most otolaryngologists resort to tubes in one to two months when antibiotics are unsuccessful in resolving a case of otitis media. Yet, in one survey, 40 percent of otolaryngologists felt that tubes were used too frequently.[7,8]

How It's Done

A child is first placed under general anesthesia. The surgeon locates the ideal spot on the eardrum for placement of the tube and makes an incision. A tiny tube is then placed through the opening. Tubes vary in size, material and design, but are basically similar. The term tympanostomy derives its meaning from the words tympanum, which is the middle ear cavity, and ostomy, which refers to any surgery in which an artificial opening is formed.

The Rationale

Doctors generally recommend tubes after antibiotics have failed to clear up a recurring earache. The hope is that tubes will:

- Reduce middle ear pressure.
- Allow fluid to drain from the middle ear.
- Restore hearing.
- Prevent permanent hearing damage.
- Prevent recurring ear infections.

Tubes are able to reduce middle ear pressure, allow fluid to drain, and improve hearing in the short term (1–3 months). But whether tubes can prevent long-term hearing loss or prevent recurrent otitis is a source of controversy. Moreover, there is a great likelihood that the underlying disease is unaffected.

Effectiveness and Complications

There is considerable controversy over the effectiveness and safety of tubes. Back in 1984, Gunnar Stickler, M.D., of the Department of Pediatrics at the Mayo Clinic, argued that there was insufficient research to justify the use of tubes. He further noted that we should, "... declare a moratorium on tube placements until solid data supporting the procedure have been reported."[9]

In the time since Dr. Stickler's remarks, numerous studies on tube placement have been conducted. The lack of encouraging results has only served to fuel the controversy. Two recent, well-designed studies at the University of Pittsburgh attempted to determine whether surgery was better than no surgery with respect to 1) the amount of time with middle ear fluid, 2) the average hearing level, and 3) the adverse effects of surgery. A review of the two studies led to the conclusion that:

- Myringotomy is an unnecessary surgical procedure.

- Children in the non-surgical group ultimately required the smallest number of surgical procedures. In other words, surgery seemed to lead to more surgery.

- Average hearing levels over a three-year period differed by less than two decibels from the surgical group to the non-surgical group. In essence, there was no significant difference in hearing.[10,11]

The third finding is especially significant since the effort to prevent hearing loss is often the sole reason for placing tubes.

Dr. Michael Pichichero and his colleagues completed a study of the complications of ears treated with tympanostomy tubes compared with those managed without surgery. Tympanosclerosis was found in the ears of 6.5 percent of the non-surgical group versus 52.3 percent of the surgical group. Tympanosclerosis is a condition where masses of hard, dense connective tissue surrounds the eardrum and bones of the middle ear. Tympanic atrophy (eardrum wasting or weakening) was found in the ears of 4.3 percent of the non-surgical group versus 40.7 percent of the surgical group. Diminished hearing was twice as common in the surgical group compared with the medical group.[12]

There were several critics of Dr. Pichichero's study who argued on various grounds. He responded in the *Pediatric Infectious Disease Journal:*

"With regard to our conclusions that tympanostomy tube insertion produces a significant incidence of tympanosclerosis and tympanic atrophy this should not be considered at all surprising. In fact, in review of the otolaryngology literature one can reasonably conclude that it has been firmly established that tympanostomy tube insertion frequently results in an increased incidence of tympanosclerosis and tympanic atrophy compared with results of medical treatment.

"In the [eight] studies cited, otolaryngology surgeons generally performed prospective evaluations in groups of children with acute otitis media or otitis media with effusion where one ear received a single tympanostomy tube surgical placement while the other ear underwent myringotomy with concomitant medical management. Follow-up varied from 2 to 7 years. The results are similar to those reported in our paper."[13]

One means to determine the effectiveness of a medical procedure is to perform a meta-analysis. A meta-analysis evaluates the data from a body of published studies, sorts out the strengths and weaknesses, and performs statistical analysis to arrive at a conclusion. Such an analysis was performed on 12 randomized controlled surgical trials going back to 1966. In their analysis, Dr. Elizabeth Bodner and her colleagues sought to answer two questions: 1) Is surgical intervention better than no surgical intervention? and 2) Is one type of surgery better than another? They concluded that the first question and, thus, the second, could not be satisfactorily answered. They wrote:

"It is disappointing that the scientific design of the twelve randomized controlled trials of the surgical management of otitis media with effusion published since 1966 was so poor that conclusions were impossible to draw from any single study . . . and results were so variable that meta-analysis was impossible."

In the introduction to this same paper, Dr. Bodner makes a very cogent statement. She writes, ". . . a more fundamental question that remains unanswered is whether otitis media is a condition that warrants intervention at all. Simply because a condition presents itself does not necessarily mean that it must be treated, particularly when natural resolution is common."

She also notes, "The unresolved debate about the most effica-cious [effective] management of otitis media with effusion is tragic given the magnitude of resources consumed and the number of children risking inappropriate or ineffective care ..."[14]

Dr. Bodner's remarks about the potential for inappropriate care bring two other important issues to the fore. The first is whether the decision to opt for tube placement—even if one presumes it is effective—is based on appropriate indications. After analyzing over 6,000 cases of children who had undergone tube placement, roughly 60 percent of the surgeries performed were considered to have equivocal or inappropriate indications. This would suggest that many such surgeries are unnecessary and that a second opin-ion should be sought whenever surgery is recommended.[15]

The second issue has undoubtedly surprised even the most pas-sionate proponents of surgery. Oxford University physicians dis-covered that 34 percent of children undergoing surgery for otitis media with effusion were actually found not to have middle ear fluid.[16]

A Note about Adenoidectomy

The use of adenoidectomy to treat middle ear fluid has also come under fire of late. A report by Jack Paradise, M.D., filed with the National Institutes of Health, summarized his study of 281 chil-dren treated with no surgery, adenoidectomy, or adenoidectomy with tonsillectomy. After two years, neither surgical group showed any advantage over the non-surgical children in the primary out-come. That is, the number of repeated episodes of middle ear fluid was not reduced by surgery when compared with no surgery.[17]

Dr. Jacob Sadé did an extensive analysis of the existing studies and arrived at this conclusion about adenoidectomy.

- The eustachian tube is not prone to obstruction in otitis media patients. There is also no evidence that adenoids obstruct the eustachian tube.

- The flow of air through the eustachian tube, as observed in inflation-deflation tests, does not show a consistent change after adenoidectomy, and the flow of mucus does not depend on the presence or absence of adenoids.

- There is no difference in the size of adenoids between normal and otitis media children. Both acute and chronic middle ear problems can exist in the absence of adenoids.

- Adenoidectomy by itself does not lead to an immediate improvement of hearing.

Dr. Sadé also cites an interesting finding reported by several ear, nose, and throat specialists—that roughly 65 percent of their patients with chronic otitis media were without adenoids, i.e., their adenoids had been previously removed. Yet, these children continued to seek care for middle ear effusion, suggesting that adenoidectomy was ineffective in managing their middle ear problems.[18]

*   *   *

Proponents of tubes can cite their own selected studies in which tubes appear to show effectiveness. But this is precisely the kind of debate that produces difficulty for parents and doctors. When presented with evidence from different sources that come to opposite conclusions, how does one make a decision? What is the right course of action?

First, we must remember Dr. Bodner's work showing that the study designs were so poor that broad conclusions were impossible. Second, when facing a procedure with inherent risks, uncertainty about any potential gains should cause us to be cautious.

Finally, recent research has shown that many children are able to avoid surgery by avoiding foods to which they test sensitive or allergic. ENT surgeon Fred Pullen, M.D., of Miami, Florida, places all children referred for tubes on a dairy-free diet. He contends that 75 percent of these children never need tubes.[19]

Similarly, Talal Nsouli, M.D., of Georgetown University Medical School, has shown clearly that surgery can be avoided when food allergies are addressed. (See Chapter 5.) Given the strong evidence for the role of food and other factors in promoting middle ear fluid, and the doubts about effectiveness of surgery, it seems reasonable to explore such options.

Even the most ardent opponents of tubes acknowledge that the procedure has value under the right circumstances. There are certainly individual cases in which surgery has been helpful. However, the decision of whether tubes (or adenoidectomy) is best for a child is clouded by the lack of sound data documenting effectiveness. I think it can be safely argued that tubes do not provide the potential for benefit that some doctors contend. Indeed, there may be a substantial number of children who receive tubes unnecessarily.

As you read through this book, you will see there are many potential ways to favorably influence the condition of the middle ear. If one chooses the surgical route, efforts should still be made to simultaneously seek the underlying cause. Individual decisions about surgery can only be made after considering all the factors specific to a given child. In this regard, I urge you to consider not only that presented here, but opposing viewpoints as well.

Chapter 4

Hearing Loss
and Delayed Development:
Myth or Reality?

Who shall decide when doctors disagree?
Alexander Pope

Parents are rightfully concerned about the prospects of otitis media leading to hearing loss in their children. The added possibility of intellectual impairment, resulting from prolonged hearing loss, has caused parents and doctors to perceive otitis media as a serious and dreaded condition that requires rigorous therapy. Yet over the years, conflicting research has made the issue of otitis media, hearing loss, and delayed development a confusing one.

Normal hearing occurs when sound waves travel from their source to the eardrum. The eardrum vibrates, setting the ear ossicles—bones of the middle ear—in motion. Vibration of the ear ossicles causes vibration of a fluid within the inner ear. This fluid passes over tiny hairlike structures that connect to nerve fibers. These fibers conduct impulses to the part of the nervous system where sound is perceived.

Proper function of the eardrum is dependent upon the pressure being equal on both sides. Equal pressure is accomplished by the eustachian tube opening and closing, according to the external pressure. Consider the pressure you feel in your ears when riding in an elevator or traveling up a mountain road. The rapid change in altitude results in a change in atmospheric pressure, causing a change in the pressure exerted on the eardrum from the outside. Swallowing or yawning generally opens the eustachian tube sufficiently to allow air to rush in or out of the middle ear, thus equalizing the internal and external pressure on the eardrum. It is these constant adjustments to the changing external environment that allow the eardrum to function normally under almost any condition. Normal function of the ear ossicles is dependent upon the same conditions. In order for them to conduct sound properly, they require an "air-filled" or aerated environment. This is also accomplished by the eustachian tube.

Any interference with the vibration of either the eardrum or middle ear ossicles can lead to a decrease in hearing acuity. This is precisely what occurs during middle ear infection or inflammation. When fluid or pus accumulates in the middle ear, pressure is exerted outward on the eardrum, causing it to be fixed and rigid. In the fluid-filled environment, the ear ossicles no longer vibrate freely. The combination of these two factors leads to to decreased *conduction* of sound waves and impaired hearing ability. Another common contributor to decreased hearing is congestion within the nasal cavity, which obstructs the opening of the eustachian tube, preventing the middle ear from being properly aerated. This leads to increased pressure within the middle ear, a feeling of fullness, and sometimes pain. The above type of hearing deficiency is known as **conductive hearing loss** and is the most common form associated with otitis media.

Another form of hearing loss is less common and more serious. It is known as **sensorineural hearing loss** and occurs when there has been residual damage to nerves and structures of the inner ear. This form of hearing loss is more likely to occur in children with chronic recurrent otitis media or otitis media that is untreated.

There is no disagreement over whether otitis media leads to temporary losses in hearing. Hearing changes in children with acute otitis media are usually short-lived, lasting only weeks to months. Children with chronic recurrent otitis media often experience hearing difficulty that is longer-lasting. Yet in most cases, the hearing impairment suffered by these children is modest and generally not sufficient even to interfere with ordinary communication.[1,2] Whether otitis media leads to permanent hearing impairment is another question.

Robert S. Mendelsohn, M.D., has long contended that ear infections do not lead to permanent hearing loss. In *The People's Doctor*, he states, "If a high percentage of untreated ear infections were to result in hearing loss, the incidence of deafness in children would be staggering, since many ear infections are undetected by the mother, undetected by a physician, inadequately treated (since not all patients take the prescribed amount of medication), and not often checked afterward to see whether they have disappeared. In some school screening tests, when children with no intervening treatment, they showed normal levels of hearing."[3]

The issues upon which some controversy rest are whether changes in hearing lead to development delays, and if so, whether the delays are permanent.

Several recent studies have suggested that there is no link between early childhood ear infections and developmental delays. Dr. Denzil Brooks, in a 1986 study of 80 children, concluded that "no correlations were found to support the hypothesis that middle ear dysfunction during the early years of schooling is causally related to poor academic achievement."[4] A study published in the journal *Pediatrics* in 1986 also found no correlation between poor academic performance and early childhood otitis media.[5]

For every study that shows no link between otitis media, hearing loss, and delayed development, there appears to be a study that confirms a link. In a review of the medical literature, Dr. C.R. Kirkwood states that "all studies reviewed show a strong correlation between otitis media and learning disabilities having several times the incidence of otitis media of controls."[6] However, in response to this argument, some researchers contend that the possibility exists that other underlying factors, common to both otitis media and learning disability, may be responsible for the correlation.*[7]

---

*For example, scientists estimate that 20 to 30 percent of children under age six have unacceptably high levels of lead in their bodies. Lead is a known inhibitor of immune function and can increase a child's suscepti-

Many studies that show an association between otitis media and developmental impairments have relied on parental recall, which is not viewed widely as a reliable means of assessment. According to one researcher, several studies dealt with children referred to a clinic *because* of academic achievement.

Even if there were evidence to support a direct link between otitis media and delayed intellectual development, the question remains whether the developmental delays are permanent. The results of a five-year follow-up of these children, published in the *British Journal of Audiology,* found that their hearing had improved substantially and their academic performance was on a par with their peers.[10]

While direct links to intellectual impairment have been difficult to prove, there is evidence of behavioral changes developing in children whose earaches are long-standing. In one study, 44 children were followed for three years after birth and assessed for cognitive and academic performance. No correlation was found between early childhood otitis media with effusion and these measures of academic achievement. However, it was learned that the children with more otitis media with effusion "... tended to be described by their teachers as less task-oriented and less able to work independently."[11] The children in this study were all in day care, which puts them at greater risk to developing otitis media. They were also socioeconomically disadvantaged, which puts them at greater risk both to otitis media and to delayed intellectual development.

Evidently, controversy still surrounds the issue of hearing loss and delayed development. The absence of a direct link is impor-

---

bility to infection. Lead also contributes to hearing problems and learning disability. It is conceivable that a percentage of children who suffer from recurrent otitis media, hearing problems, and learning problems do so as a result of lead toxicity. (To my knowledge, this relationship has not been thoroughly studied.) A principal cause of lead toxicity in children is inhalation and ingestion of lead-laden dust from leaded house paint. This is a very serious problem. See chapter 7 for more information on lead.

tant because some doctors base their rationale for treatment (especially surgical) on the "threat" of potential permanent hearing loss and delayed development. On this, J.L. Paradise, M.D. comments "What seems *not* reasonable, however, is to subject largely asymptomatic infants or young children with middle-ear effusions to surgical intervention relatively early in the course of their illness, i.e., less than two to three months after onset, invoking as sole justification the fear of later developmental handicaps."[12]

At the University of Pittsburgh, in perhaps the largest ongoing study of its kind, Dr. Paradise has found little evidence of developmental delay occurring as result of otitis media.[13]

This does not imply that children with otitis media should go untreated or that those with hearing loss should be ignored. Despite the existence of conflicting evidence, audiologists have expressed alarm over the growing number of preschool children who are minimally hearing impaired. Many feel that recurrent otitis media impacts adversely upon learning, speech, behavior, and even interaction with peers.

According to Lilian Rojas, Ph.D., a speech, hearing, and language specialist, aphasiologist, and international consultant to educational institutions, all persons who work with children, from physicians to educators, must be made aware of the potential problems facing children with hearing deficits. Dr. Rojas cites evidence that there are critical stages of development that can be delayed by the presence of persistent middle ear effusion. She states that in some children with middle ear effusion, hearing may fall within the normal decibel range but the quality of sound perception may suffer. Hearing may seem "normal," but some sounds perceived by the child are distorted. For instance, the ability to distinguish between different consonants may be impaired, which leads to problems with reading and language.

The children most adversely affected by the triad of otitis media, hearing loss, and delayed development are those living in low socioeconomic conditions (although the effects are by no means restricted to these children). This includes the growing number of children living with a single parent and those of immigrant parents. In both groups, the financial resources, access to good health care, availability of nutritious food and nutrition information is severely restricted. In immigrant populations, parents are often uneducated about the need to treat otitis media and the consequences that may follow if hearing loss is persistent.

Sadly, many children with hearing impairment are labeled early in life as learning disabled or unintelligent, much like "deaf" persons were labeled in the past. Proper treatment and monitoring of young children with middle ear effusion is important if we are to effectively address their needs. The underlying factors leading up to otitis media must also be addressed. These are discussed in the following chapter.

Chapter 5

Causes of Childhood
Ear Infections

By definition, otitis media is a disease of the ears. Fluid accumulates in the middle ear, pressure develops in the middle ear, and pain occurs in the middle ear. Quite naturally then, doctors should directly treat the ears by whatever means possible. Or should they? One great weakness in modern medical practice is failure to view the patient as a whole. When a problem arises in one area of the body, this is often the only area that receives attention. This is why antibiotics and surgery are used with such great frequency.

What happens if we ask the question, "What has occurred to render the child's defenses unable to cope with a viral or bacterial insult?" In epidemics of strep throat, up to 60 percent of people are considered "carriers." That is, they have positive strep cultures, but do not get sick. If one tests healthy children in an elementary school classroom, he might discover that up to 40 percent of them culture positive for mycoplasma in their lungs. Yet, these children are not sick. In studies of stress and infection, those under high stress are much more likely to become sick than those under low stress, even though both may culture positive for bacteria such as strep. What is unique about the individuals who remain well?

I am convinced the difference lies in immune defenses, or host defenses. In 1994, we reviewed over one thousand research papers in writing *Beyond Antibiotics* (North Atlantic Books, Berkeley, California). It became clear that the immune system could be positively or negatively influenced by at least six factors:

- Diet

- Nutrition

- Lifestyle

- Environment

- Neuromusculoskeletal factors

- Psychological factors

Imbalance in one or more areas might tip the scales in favor of the bacteria or virus. Maintaining balance in these areas often allows one to remain well despite exposure to bacteria or viruses. The principles set forth in *Beyond Antibiotics* have now been used successfully by hundreds of thousands of patients of all ages around the world. The growing consensus is that by improving host defenses one can reduce the rate of infection and reduce reliance on antibiotic drugs.

Can the same principles be applied to childhood otitis media? Can the principles be applied to prevention as well as treatment? Since the first edition of *Childhood Ear Infections* was published, parents and physicians from many nations have written or called. The overwhelmingly positive feedback shows that we can reduce the suffering from middle ear problems and improve overall health and vitality.

Otitis media is an inflammation of the middle ear. All the events that occur in the middle ear—swelling, pain, infection, complications—are important and must be addressed. However, these events may only be the sequel to events that occur elsewhere in the body. Killing bacteria may, at times, be necessary. But as you read this chapter, keep in mind that optimizing immune function is highly desirable regardless of age or condition.

The cause of otitis media is not fully understood. There may, in fact, be no singular cause of the disease. What probably occurs is a multiplicity of events that interact to take advantage of lowered immune function, underdeveloped eustachian tube muscles, respiratory congestion, excessive mucus production, nutritional inadequacy, or any number of other factors. In this section, I present a synthesis of the major contributing factors in middle ear inflammation. In each case, prevention and treatment solutions are available that take advantage of our understanding of the causes presented here.

The four main causes of otitis media are:*

- Allergy and Environmental Sensitivity.
- Infection.
- Mechanical Obstruction.
- Nutrient Insufficiency.

Allergy and Environmental Sensitivity

Allergy is called the great masquerader because it can contribute to and mimic many illnesses with which we don't usually associate allergy.[2] From recurrent colds to bronchitis, bedwetting to headaches, enlarged tonsils to diarrhea, allergy can play a significant role. To children with recurrent middle ear infection, allergy is indeed the "great masquerader." Allergy can contribute to swollen tonsils, nasal and sinus congestion, swollen mucous membranes of the eustachian tube, and ultimately, fluid in the middle ear. In some children, the persistence of allergy leads to the chronic buildup of a very viscous and mucoid fluid in the middle ear.

Not all children with allergies develop middle ear problems, and not all children with middle ear problems have them because of allergies. But in children whose earaches are due to allergy, neglecting to treat the allergy (or the underlying factors that lead to the development of allergies) often results in recurrent infections.

Evidence demonstrating the role of allergy in middle ear prob-

---

*In 1976, W. Leonard Draper, M.D. stated that childhood otitis media has multiple causes, and multiple phases. He listed among the causes allergy, infection, and mechanical blockage. Since 1976, our understanding of nutrition has expanded substantially making it clear that nutritional factors also play an important role in the development of otitis media.[1]

lems has been steadily accumulating over the past four decades. A study of 540 children by W. Leonard Draper, M.D., showed that secretory otitis media was more than twice as frequent in allergic children than in non-allergic children.[3] Draper also noted, in a study of 100 allergic children, that approximately 50 percent had fluid in the ears.[4] Poor eustachian tube function—believed to be one of the prime factors leading to the development of middle ear infection— has been found to occur in almost one-third of allergic children.[5]

No one is certain of the percentage of children with allergy-related otitis media. The available evidence suggests that from 11 to 85 percent of cases have an allergic component.[6,7] Dr. L.Q. Pang, Clinical Professor of Surgery at the University of Hawaii Medical School, insists that allergy plays a significant role in otitis media. He states that "a large percentage of chronic suppurative otitis media with a central perforation [of the eardrum] is due to an allergy."[8]

Dr. D.C. Heiner and his associates report in the *Annals of Allergy* that "childhood otitis media may be solely, or partially due to food allergy." He goes on to stress that much of the tonsilar or adenoid swelling, and even upper airway obstruction, may be caused or aggravated by food allergies.[9] Doris Rapp, M.D., author of numerous books on childhood allergy, states that avoidance of the major offending food items, or indoor problematic allergens, can help many patients with otitis media. More importantly, she says that "by eliminating the cause of the medical problem [through allergy management], it is often possible to obviate [eliminate] not only the need for surgery, but also the necessity to mask the patient's symptoms with medications."[10]

Dr. George Shambaugh, Professor Emeritus of Otolaryngology at Northwestern University and former president of the American Academy of Otolaryngology, gave an address in 1982 entitled, "Serous Otitis: Are Tubes the Answer?" In his lecture, he addresses the question of allergy, stating, "Although allergies in children are often hard to identify by the usual allergy scratch tests, I've found that a program of allergic management with attention to hidden or delayed-in-onset food allergy helps me manage recurrent ear problems in children. Moreover, my results with allergy management are far better than those obtained by putting children on prolonged courses of antibiotics, and relying on tubes to clear up the condition."[11]

If allergies are a factor in middle ear infection, there should be evidence that shows a capacity for allergens to cause adverse changes in the middle ear and eustachian tube. We also would expect children with allergy-related earaches to improve with some form of allergy management.

Allergens can cause direct changes within the middle ear and eustachian tube. Dr. Robert O'Conner and his colleagues have observed that significant and rapid pressure changes take place in the middle ear of children when their nasal passages are exposed to allergens.[12] Other scientists have found that allergens can cause obstruction of the eustachian tube that lasts for up to 14 days. Often, a blocked eustachian tube can be encouraged to open by swallowing, but in cases where tube blockage occurs because of allergy, swallowing appears to have little impact. These findings suggest an allergic basis for eustachian tube obstruction and possibly for the development of middle ear disease.[13]

The response of allergic children with otitis media to proper allergy management can be swift and dramatic. Dr. John P. McGovern and his associates studied 512 children with allergy and middle ear problems. Using careful allergy management, these doctors reported good or excellent results with 97 percent of the children.[14] A 1982 report in the *International Journal of Pediatric Otorhinolaryngology* revealed that elimination diets—for children who tested positive for foods— were useful in the treatment of otitis media. A significant finding in this study of 67 children was that "fewer operations were needed in the treatment of patients with elimination diets."[15]

Despite these and other studies, many doctors have been slow to consider the role of food intolerance or allergy in middle ear problems. Today, the results of a study by Dr. Talal M. Nsouli and his colleagues at Georgetown University School of Medicine cannot be overlooked. Dr. Nsouli's group tested 104 children with recurrent middle ear problems for food allergy and discovered 81 to be allergic. After eliminating offending foods for 16 weeks, 86 percent experienced "significant amelioration" of their middle ear problem. When offending foods were reintroduced, 94 percent of the children got worse—their middle ear fluid returned.

The most common offending foods were:

- Cow's milk products (38%)
- Wheat (33%)
- Egg white (25%)
- Peanut (20%)
- Soy (17%)

Other foods such as corn, orange, tomato, and chicken were found as well, though less commonly. Most children were found to be allergic to more than one food. In fact, 81 percent of the children were allergic to two to four foods.

Another key to the study, children were kept off offending foods for 16 weeks. This study showed that many elimination diets that last only two to three weeks may not be long enough to notice an effect. It may be necessary to keep the child off allergenic foods for 11 to 16 weeks.

Dr. Nsouli's group concluded, "The possibility of food allergy should be considered in all patients with recurrent serous otitis media and a diligent search for the putative food allergen made for proper diagnostic and therapeutic intervention." Similar to the previous study, Dr. Nsouli's group reported that "We were able to avoid surgery in the majority of the patients who avoided the offending foods." Thus, it seems safe to say that the existence of food allergy or food intolerance should be thoroughly assessed in children with chronic middle ear problems.[16]

What Is an Allergy?

Doctors disagree on the extent to which allergies play a role in middle ear problems. Many allergists contend that what people call allergies today are not really allergies. They argue that "true" allergy requires an IgE reaction. IgE stands for immunoglobulin E, which is a protein commonly produced by white blood cells during aller-

Figure 2		
Research Linking Ear Infection to Allergy		
Researcher/Journal	**Year**	**Allergy Type**
Draper, *Clinical Ecology*	1976	Food-Airborne
Shambaugh, American Academy of Otolaryngology (Lecture)	1982	Food-Airborne
Mogi, *Acta Otorhinolaryngology Belgium*	1983	Food-Airborne
Friedman, *Journal of Allergy and Clinical Immunology*	1983	Food-Airborne
Bernstein, *American Journal of Otolaryngology*	1983	Airborne
Rapp, *American Journal of Otolaryngology*	1984	Food-Airborne
Heiner, *Annals of Allergy*	1984	Food-Airborne
Kraemer, *Clinical Reviews in Allergy*	1984	Airborne
Ackerman, *Journal of Allergy and Clinical Immunology*	1984	Airborne
Hurst, *Otolaryngol Head Neck Surg*	1990	Food-Airborne
Nsouli, *Ann Allergy*	1994	Food

gic reactions. Much contemporary research shows that the body reacts adversely to foreign substances in a variety of ways—not only through IgE. In fact, IgE reactions play a role in the earaches of perhaps only 15 percent of children described as allergic on the basis of clinical and laboratory evidence.[17] Dr. E. Pastorello has found a surprisingly high incidence of food intolerance that is not related to IgE.[18]

To speak accurately of the way in which people adversely react to substances with which they come in contact, we have to use the terms allergy and hypersensitivity. *Allergy* is defined as an adverse response brought about by exposure to a substance in the environment—called an allergen. These reactions occur because the immune system recognizes the substance(s) as a threat and goes into an attack mode to eliminate the threat. *Hypersensitivity* (the term intolerance is sometimes used) is an adverse reaction to a substance for any other reason.

An example of true allergy is a child who develops a runny nose, watery eyes, sneezing, and stuffiness when exposed to ragweed pollen. When the blood is tested in such children, IgE antibodies are often elevated, along with an elevation in the white cells called eosinphils. Examples of hypersensitivity include adverse reactions to two common food additives—monosodium glutamate (MSG) and sulfites. MSG—a substance to which many people are sensitive—is used widely as a flavor enhancer. Sulfites are a family of compounds used to preserve the whiteness of foods such as sugar, flour, baking powder, and dried fruit.

Hypersensitivity reactions to foods or additives are frequently due to nutritional deficiency or problems with improperly functioning enzymes. For example, scientists have observed that many MSG-sensitive individuals who are given B6 are no longer sensitive to MSG.[19] This suggest that the enzyme needed to properly metabolize MSG is enhanced by B6. In individuals who are not B6-supplemented, ingested MSG builds up in the system rather than being processed and eliminated efficiently.

The enzyme that helps to break down excess sulfite happens to be dependent upon the micro-trace element molybdenum.[20] Deficiency of molybdenum can impair the enzyme, which leads to a build-up of sulfite in the body, which leads to symptoms. The symptoms persist until either the sulfites are eliminated from the diet, or molybdenum is added to the diet. Sulfites can aggravate or cause upper respiratory reactions in sensitive individuals. I've even observed cases of sulfite-related otitis media.

How Allergies May Contribute to Middle Ear Problems

- Allergens may trigger collapse or narrowing of the eustachian tube. This interferes with normal opening and closing, thereby reducing ventilation of the middle ear.

- Allergens may cause swollen tonsils or adenoids, leading to reduced elimination (or drainage) of lymph fluid (see Heiner). This mechanically obstructs the eustachian tube opening.

- Allergens can initiate excessive production of mucus and serous fluid. This results in reduced ventilation of the middle ear, reduced drainage of the middle ear, and slowed movement of white blood cells to the site of infection.

- Allergens, especially food allergens, can inhibit the white blood cells' ability to digest and destroy bacteria.

This is a fairly simple assessment of the way in which allergy contributes to middle ear problems. The true mechanism is not well understood, and at this time, is considered theoretical.

Testing for Food Allergy

There are several methods available to test for allergy or sensitivity to food. No single test is 100 percent accurate. Each test conveys slightly different information. Below is a very brief discussion of commonly used tests. Recognize that the field of allergy as well as the concept of what constitutes an adverse food reaction are evolving, and that information presented here will likely change as we learn more.

Blood Test for IgE. IgE is an antibody that is produced in response to foreign substances (usually). IgE (immunoglobulin E) responses usually occur within minutes to hours after consuming a food. Thus, the test is useful in detecting immediate hypersensitivity reactions. A drawback is that it does not measure delayed reactions to food nor does it measure intolerance to food that is not mediated by the immune system.

Blood Test for IgG. IgG reactions generally occur over a longer period of time and are responsible for delayed reactions. There are two primary types of tests—total IgG and IgG4. Proponents of both make strong arguments for the value of one over the other. IgG tests do not measure immediate reactions and, therefore, do not detect reactions that occur within minutes to hours of consuming a food. Some doctors believe a combination of IgE and IgG blood tests gives a comprehensive look at food reactivity.

Provocation/Neutralization. This is an office-based test where the doctor injects a tiny amount of a suspected allergen under the skin and observes for a reaction. The reactions can sometimes be dramatic when foods to which a child is sensitive are introduced. When an allergen is found, the doctor then introduces a tiny neutralizing dose that will eliminate the symptoms. This dose is then used to treat the allergic response. Dr. Doris Rapp of Buffalo, New York has extensive experience with this technique and has published several papers and books in which this is discussed. (See Is *This Your Child*, New York, Quill, 1991.)

Lactulose/Mannitol Test. Doctors increasingly recognize that increased intestinal permeability, or leaky gut, is at the root of food intolerance in some children. Moreover, when a child continues to consume a food to which she is sensitive, the leaky gut condition often worsens. This may lead to development of sensitivity to additional foods. The lactulose/mannitol urine test measures the degree to which two simple ingested sugars are absorbed into the body.

The journal *Food Allergy in Pediatrics* recently reviewed a study comparing the lactulose/mannitol ratio in children with food allergies to that of normal children. They concluded, "The intestinal permeability test for the diagnosis of food allergies seems to be a sensitive and noninvasive test that is well suited to the pediatric practice."[21] The test can also identify absorption problems. If leaky gut syndrome exists, dietary and nutritional strategies aimed at repair are necessary.

The Most Common Offenders

Allergy and hypersensitivity reactions can be triggered by virtually any substance to which a child is exposed. There are two major categories of substances which initiate these reactions—food and airborne. Within these categories, there are some substances that contribute to otitis media more frequently than others. This reduces the pursuit of potential offenders from thousands to only a handful. In general, food allergy/hypersensitivity contributes more to otitis media than does airborne. However, each category contains important offenders.

Food Allergy and Hypersensitivity

In a study of 1,000 patients with food allergy, Dr. Frederic Speer found that milk, chocolate, cola, corn, citrus, and egg were the most common allergens. Milk allergies were especially common in children under two.[22] Of all foods, cow's milk and other dairy products are probably the number one contributor to childhood ear problems. These and other common allergens implicated in otitis media are listed below.

- Dairy products, including milk, butter, cheese, yogurt, cottage cheese, cow's milk formula, and *ice cream*.

- Wheat, including not only bread and cereal, but anything that contains wheat such as gravies, crackers, and cookies.

- Eggs and anything containing eggs.

- Chocolate.

- Citrus, especially oranges and orange juice.

- Corn, or anything containing corn, such as corn flakes.

- Soy. This is especially a problem with infant formula. Dr. William Crook states that 25 percent of infants with a milk allergy develop an allergy to soy.

- Peanuts and other nuts. Peanut butter is a great favorite among children and a frequent contributor to childhood health problems.

- Shellfish.

- Sugar.

- Yeast.

Food allergy can be a nemesis because the offenders hide among a variety of foods children consume every day. In many cases, the foods to which a child is allergic or sensitive are those that she eats the most. Commonly, children are addicted to foods. The cravings can be so intense that a child will refuse to eat unless her "favorite" food is given at mealtime. I've seen this occur with cheese, crackers, milk, peanut butter, and virtually all items on the above list.

Foods that are consumed every day, or several times a day, can lead to the development of allergy of hypersensitivity to that food. Children with a daily diet that consists of only a handful of items are at risk to developing food allergies. I am reminded of a five-year-old girl named April who suffered from recurrent middle ear problems that did not respond to antibiotic treatment. When I asked about April's favorite foods the mother and father looked at one another and laughed. "We call her our little cheese curd," quipped the mother. "Why?" I asked with a grin. The mother said, "She loves cheese so much. In fact, at home we tie a cheese cutter to a string and hang it around her neck. That way, she can get a piece whenever she likes."

It didn't take a great leap of logic to deduce that removing cheese from little April's diet might be the solution. In fact, here is a good example of a child who has food allergy or intolerance, yet is driven by almost addiction-like urges to consume the food that is, to her, most damaging. In April's case, removing all dairy products, especially cheese, eventually solved her problem.

In chapter 2, I described how antibiotic use contributes to the development of food allergies by eradicating beneficial intestinal bacteria. In one study, *all* children suffering from symptoms of food allergies had evidence of deficiencies of *Lactobacilli* and *Bifidobacteria* in the intestinal tract. They also had and overgrowth of other enteric bacteria.[23] When the intestinal bacteria are restored through supplementation, food allergies frequently improve. (See chapter 6.)

Airborne Allergy and Sensitivity

Airborne substances easily contribute to upper respiratory and ear problems because they are in constant contact with the mucous membranes of these parts of the body. In children who are not allergic, airborne allergens usually don't cause much trouble (although one family of indoor air pollutants, discussed later, can cause significant mucous membrane irritation even in non-allergic children).

The average adult spends only one hour per day outdoors. The average child spends only slightly more time outdoors, especially in northern climates. Because the vast *quantity* of air children breath is indoor air, it is essential that the indoor air be of good *quality*. Unfortunately, the indoor air in most American homes, schools, and offices is full of contaminants. These pollutants are contributing to an increase in chronic health complaints in both children and adults. The most common indoor air pollutants are:

- Cigarette smoke.
- Volatile organic compounds.
- Pollen.
- Carbon monoxide.
- Animal dander.

- House dust.
- Mold.
- Fungi.
- Sulfur dioxide.
- Bacteria.

The most pernicious airborne irritant in otitis media is sidestream **cigarette smoke**. Dr. Michael Kraemer and his colleagues reported in the *Journal of the American Medical Association* in 1983 that the incidence of otitis media with effusion increases nearly three-fold when a child is exposed to two or more household smokers. When exposed to smoke from more than three packs of cigarettes per day, the risk increases four-fold.[24]

Children of smoking parents are admitted to hospitals nearly 28 percent more often than children of non-smoking parents. Those exposed to second-hand cigarette smoke also lose more days to sickness from respiratory ailments (which is significant because 50 percent of all earaches follow an upper respiratory problem of some type).[25] See Figure 3.

There are probably many reasons why cigarette smoke causes an increase in childhood ear infections. Recent evidence suggests that the level of vitamin E is lower in the lungs of smokers than in the lungs of non-smokers. Vitamin E is an important antioxidant nutrient that protects cell membranes from free-radical damage. Free radicals are highly reactive chemical species that cause destruction of cells through chain reactions. Scientists estimate that one puff of sidestream (second-hand) cigarette smoke contains up to one hundred-trillion or 100,000,000,000,000 (10^{14}) free radicals.[27] When the delicate lining of the respiratory tract is exposed to the large number of free radicals found in cigarette smoke (see Fig-

	Children's Restricted Activity Days	Children's Bed-Disability Days
No Smokers in Home (control)	—	—
1 Smoker in Home	+ 7 percent	+ 14 percent
2 or More Smokers in Home	+ 29 percent	+ 29 percent
45 or More Cigarettes per Day	+ 46 percent	+ 43 percent

Figure 3
Comparative "Sick Days" Among Children of Smoking and Nonsmoking Households

(Adapted from Bonham and Wilson, 1981)[26]

Figure 4
Principal Constituents of Cigarette Smoke*

Particles:

tar	pyrene
nicotine	benzo (a) pyrene
perylene	benzo (b) pyrene
benzo (ghi) perylene	dibenz (a,j) anthracene
fluoranthene	dibenz (ah) anthracene
benzo (a) fluorene	ideno (2,3-ed) chrysene
benzo (b) fluorene	benz (a) anthracene
cadmium	anthanthrene
phenol	benzo (b/k/j) fluoranthrene

Gases and Vapors:

water	acrolein
carbon monoxide	formaldehyde
ammonia	toluene
carbon dioxide	acetone
nitrogen oxides	polonium-210
hydrogen cyanide	

Source: U.S. National Research Council, Committee on Indoor Pollutants, 1981 p. iv–101.[28]

*Many airborne pollutants are absorbed as freely, or more freely through the lungs than through the intestines or skin. Therefore, breathing some of these substances is not much different from eating or drinking them.

---

ure 4), significant demands are placed on the antioxidant defense mechanism of the respiratory tract, leading to vitamin E deficiency.

Vitamin C is another member of the antioxidant defense system designed to protect the delicate lining of our cell membranes from injury. Cigarette smoke causes vitamin C to be excreted more rapidly in the urine of smokers and presumably in the urine of children exposed to second-hand smoke as well.

The depletion of protective antioxidant nutrients by exposure to smoke is significant since sidestream smoke is often more toxic than inhaled smoke (especially when filtered cigarettes are used). The reduced antioxidant levels result in changes in the cells lining the respiratory tract, leading to a reduced ability to remove allergens, bacteria, and viruses. The lining of the middle ear cavity consists of cells very similar to those lining the lungs and other parts of the respiratory tract. The irritants found in smoke cause much the same damage to the lining of the middle ear as they do to the lungs and nasal passages.

Sidestream smoke has been shown to paralyze cilia within the respiratory tract. The lining of the middle ear and respiratory tract consists of a layer of stratified, column-shaped cells covered with tiny hairlike cilia that help remove allergens and microbes from the middle ear. During exposure to cigarette smoke, the cilia are destroyed or impaired. This reduces the ability of the middle ear to remove invading microbes and allergens. The consequences include middle ear effusion and infection.

House dust is another common airborne offender that can contribute to otitis media. It contributes to illness because of its ability to carry tremendous numbers of allergens, toxicants, and microbes. House dust is a complex mixture of hundreds of items including lint, snips of hair, oils, animal dander (including human skin), and particles of textiles from rugs, bedding, furniture, drapes, carpet padding, clothing, and pillows. One teaspoon of house dust can contain from 5 to 10 million microbes—including some very nasty bacteria and viruses. After a short incubation period, the numbers can rise into the billions.

One of the most common irritants found in household dust is the house dust mite. According to G. W. Wharton, many people are more allergic to mites than to other house dust components.[29] This tiny arthropod feeds on human skin and resides in mattresses, carpeting, draperies, and any household item that harbors dust. Vacuum cleaners left standing with a partially full bag often serve as hotels in which millions of house dust mites eat, reproduce, live, and grow old.

House dust is also a principal source of lead, cadmium, and other heavy metals. In studies of cognitive function in children, Dr. Robert Thatcher and his associates showed that serum and tissue lead and cadmium levels in children correlated directly with the level of house dust. Apparently, the children come in contact with heavy metals through the dust that collects on their hands during play. The dust is then transferred to mouth by normal hand-to-mouth activity. In these studies, lead and cadmium were shown to have adverse effect on verbal IQ and performance IQ.[30] Lead and cadmium are also known to have an adverse effect on immune function. Reduction of house of house dust is one important element in controlling exposure to these metals. (Incidentally, children with adequate levels of zinc appear to be partially insulated against the adverse effects of cadmium, while those with adequate calcium are insulated against the adverse effects of lead.)

In the average home, roughly 40 pounds of house dust are produced annually. It is a significant problem for infants and toddlers because they spend the better part of their day crawling and shuffling around on the floor. Dust is further circulated by common forced-air furnaces and vacuum cleaners. (See chapter 7 on prevention.) To the allergic child, the continual dose of allergens and microbes in house dust creates significant upper respiratory irritation and contributes to chronic upper respiratory disease, otitis media, tonsillitis, and rhinitis. Children who are not "allergic" may still suffer, due to the presence of such large numbers of agents that can potentially challenge the immune system.

A fairly recent addition to the family of indoor air pollutants/respiratory irritants is a group of chemicals called **volatile organic compounds** (VOC). VOC are organic chemicals that evaporate at temperatures of 32 degrees Fahrenheit and higher. They are constituents of common household items. Among these are cleaning compounds, newsprint, mothballs, and even furniture. Building materials are one of the greatest sources of VOC. These include particle board, paint, varnish, caulking compounds, carpeting, vinyl floor covering, and more.

We are only beginning to understand the scope of this problem. In 1985, the EPA studied 11 VOC's indoors. Their findings revealed unacceptable levels of compounds such as benzene, trichloroethane, and styrene—all of which are not only membrane irritants but carcinogens as well. Levels of all tested compounds were higher indoors than outdoors. The home's age or location seemed to have no bearing on pollutant levels. From new urban homes to old rural homes, the problem of volatile pollutants was similar.[31]

In Baton Rouge, Houston, and Greensborough, the EPA measured levels of 32 volatile chemicals and found all to be higher in the indoor air than in the outdoor air.[32] Public access buildings such as schools, office buildings, and day care facilities are often among the worst offenders. In a Washington, D.C., home for the elderly, 350 different volatile chemicals were identified *in the air*. Of these, 35 were found at all locations tested, and 12 were known carcinogens or mutagens.[33]

The air quality in homes is also among the worst. In Oak Ridge, Tennessee, federal scientists monitored 40 homes for the presence of organic vapors in the air. During the study period, they identified between 20 and 150 solvents and other volatile chemicals in the indoor air of *each structure*! Only 10 were found in the outdoor air.[34] These and similar studies reveal that indoor air pollution is a serious and growing problem.

Where Do Indoor Air Pollutants Come From?

Indoor air pollutants are generated from building materials and household products. Almost every aspect of our lives involves the use of synthetic materials. These synthetic materials release vapors that, over time, contribute to ill health in a large number of people.

Carpeting is one of the worst offenders. Carpeting is comprised of synthetic fibers derived from petroleum. At various stages of processing, chemicals are added to carpet to make it stain-resistant and fire-resistant. Insecticides and fungicides are often added to carpeting to protect it against mold, mildew, and fungus. These

Figure 5	
Summary of Other Studies of Indoor Air Pollutants	
Molhave	Found elevated levels of benzene & toluene in 39 dwellings.
Jarke	Found increased concentration of organics in 34 Chicago homes.
Leberet	Concluded that 35 of 35 organics had mean indoor levels greater than outdoor levels in 134 tested homes. Seven of these indoor levels exceeded outdoor levels by 10 times. Tobacco smoking was correlated with increase of 10 organics.
Seifert	Measured 15 homes in Berlin; all had increased levels of toluene(*) and xylene from printed material.
Gammage	Detected gasoline vapors in 40 Tennessee homes, most with attached garages.

35,36,37,38,39

Note: Many early monitoring studies of indoor pollutants have been done in Europe. Those conducted in American homes yield similar results. Presently, European governments have taken the lead in reducing the indoor contaminants in the home. The U.S. government has made little progress in this regard, evidenced by the relaxed standards regarding formaldehyde in building materials.

(*) Toluene, a solvent that is carcinogen and well-known mucous membrane irritant, is the most common airborne pollutant isolated in all studies.

chemicals are highly toxic and highly irritating. What's worse, their vapors are released from the carpeting as the carpet ages. The "new carpet" smell is actually a chemical soup that wafts its way through the air. When carpeting is cleaned by professional cleaning services, more toxic compounds are added. Naphtha, a known carcinogen, is often used in the cleaning process. In addition, insecticides and stainproofing agents are applied during the cleaning.

Formaldehyde is a familiar indoor air pollutant. It is found in everything from cosmetics to clothing. One of the richest sources of formaldehyde is the waferboard used in the walls and subflooring of almost all new homes.

Old newspapers stored indoors can outgas toxic vapors for months. The printing ink contains a complex mixture of chemicals including toluene and xylene. Fuel used for heating can cause problems as well. Children in homes where wood stoves are used suffer from more respiratory ailments than children in homes where wood stoves are not used.[40] The list of sources of volatile pollutants is almost endless.

How Volatile Indoor Air Pollutants Contribute to Ear Infections

Most cases of otitis media with effusion share a common characteristic—inflammation of the mucous membrane of the middle ear and/or eustachian tube. Moreover, otitis media is frequently preceded by inflammation of the upper respiratory tract. These delicate tissues, while possessing some form of protection, are susceptible to the continuous presence of irritants in the air.

As discussed above, the vapors often found in indoor air are common constituents of the building materials used in the construction of homes, offices, and schools. When the vapors of building materials were analyzed, it was found that as high as *80 percent were known mucous membrane irritants*.[41] In other words, the items used to build and furnish our homes, schools, day care centers, and offices are replete with invisible, often odorless gases that can initiated inflammation of the middle ear (also eyes, nose, throat, and lungs). At first, constant exposure to even low levels of these airborne gases overwhelms the antioxidant defense system. As expo-

Figure 6
**Examples of Organic Compound Types
and Potential Indoor Sources**

Pollutant Type	Example	Indoor Sources
Aliphatic hydrocarbons	Propane, butane hexane, limonene	Cooking and heating fuels, aerosol propellants, cleaning compounds, refrigerants, lubricants, flavoring agents, perfume base
Halogenated hydrocarbons	Methyl chloroform, methylene chloride, PCBs	Aerosol propellants, fumigants, pesticides, refrigerants, and degreasing, dewaxing and dry cleaning solvents
Aromatic hydrocarbons	Benzene, toluene, xylenes	Paints, varnishes, glues, enamels, lacquers, cleaners
Alcohols	Ethanol, methanol	Window cleaners, paint thinners, cosmetics, adhesives human breath
Ketones	Acetone	Lacquers, varnishes, polish removers, adhesives
Aldehydes	Formaldehyde, nonanal	Fungicides, germicides, disinfectants, artificial and permanent-press textiles, paper, particle boards cosmetics, flavoring agents, etc.

From *Indoor Air and Human Health*, by R.B. Gammage and S.V. Kaye. Copyright 1985, Lewis Publishers, Inc., Chelsea, MI, p. 391. Used with permission.[42]

sure continues, inflammatory and immune changes occur that can contribute to ongoing respiratory and middle ear complaints.

This category of indoor air pollutants has become serious only since the mid-1970s, because of the increase in tighter, energy-efficient homes, coupled with rapid increase in the use of synthetic materials. Ironically, the incidence of otitis media has increased dramatically during the same period. While it is difficult to prove a link between indoor air pollutants and otitis media, it is very likely that these volatile pollutants have contributed to some of the upper respiratory irritation that often creates susceptibility to middle ear problems. The constant presence of airborne irritants also may impede the recovery of middle ear problems due to other causes.

Doris Rapp, M.D., a Fellow of the American Academy of Allergy and Immunology, has pioneered the study and treatment of environmental illness in children. Her work has appeared in medical journals and in best selling books such as *Is This Your Child* and *Sick Schools, Sick Kids, Sick Teachers.* She has shown clearly that environmental factors can be at the root of almost any physical or behavioral condition in children. Moreover, she chronicles the declining air quality in both the indoor and outdoor environment.

Her experience treating thousands of children has led her to the conclusion that middle ear problems can be triggered by exposure to mold, pollen, food, chemicals, dust or any combination of these. Dr. Rapp emphasizes the concept of **total load** as an important factor in development of symptoms. For example, on a given day, exposure to mold or pollen may not trigger symptoms. But if a sensitive child is consuming an allergenic food, is under stress, and is also exposed to mold and pollen, the total load may overwhelm their threshold of tolerance and they develop symptoms. Any combination of stressors or environmental agents can contribute to the total load.

To determine whether your child might be reacting to food or environmental substance, Dr. Rapp suggests that you look for changes in five characteristics. She calls these "The Big Five." They are:

- Pulse (increase)

- Breathing (shallow, rapid, decrease in peak flow)

- Appearance (red ears, watery eyes, puffy eyes, etc.)

- Behavior (crying, biting, hitting, anger, rage, etc.)

- Handwriting (any changes)

Middle ear problems in children have risen sharply in the past two decades. This, coupled with the questioned effectiveness of antibiotics and surgery, should cause any parent or doctor to take a serious look at the role of allergy and environmental insult.

Infection

Under certain conditions, bacteria present in the upper respiratory tract find their way up the eustachian tube into the middle ear. Once in the middle ear chamber, they contribute to the damaging events with which we usually associate infection. When middle ear fluid is cultured for bacteria, the most common bacteria found are *Haemophilus influenzae* and *Streptococcus pneumoniae*. These are called *pathogenic* organisms, which refers to their ability to produce disease. Cases of otitis media in which *S. pneumoniae* is involved tend to occur with severe pain and fever, but more commonly affect both ears.[43,44]

In a report of bacteria found in middle ear fluid from a total of 3,583 children from three countries, Dr. J.O. Klein observed the presence of either *S.pneumoniae* (35 percent) or *H. influenzae* (20 percent) in a total of 55 percent of cases.[45] During a period from 1980 to 1985, other investors found that *S. pneumoniae* and *H. influenzae* comprised 50.7 percent of bacteria isolated from the middle ear fluid of their patients (29.8 and 20.9 percent respectively).[46]

One of the largest and most recent studies concerning bacteria in middle ear fluid was conducted at the University of Pittsburgh. After examining the fluid of 4,589 middle ears, only 22 percent were found to contain harmful bacteria such as *S. pneumoniae* and *H. influenzae*.[47] Based on other analyses, only about 11 percent of culture-positive middle ear fluid contain enough bacteria to be considered an infection (> 1000 colony forming units).[48] Therefore, according to one estimate, only about two to three percent of these fluid-filled middle ears had *sufficient quantities* of bacteria to be considered an infection.

Much attention has been given to an article published in 1995 showing that 77 percent of middle ear fluid samples contained bacterial DNA.[49] This single article will undoubtedly lead to more antibiotic prescribing. Yet, it suffers from the same weaknesses as previous studies and has been harshly criticized because the mere presence of bacterial DNA does not signify that bacteria are causing the problem. Indeed, the presence of bacteria does not imply cause.

Viral infection of the respiratory tract has been found in about 46 percent of children with acute otitis media. Viruses have been found in middle ear fluid in 8 to 25 percent of such children. When viruses occur along with bacteria, the illness seems to be more difficult to resolve.[50]

Yeast, such as *Candida albicans,* have also been found in middle ears. In one study, yeast infection of the middle ear was found in all treatment-resistant children. The antifungal drug ketoconazole was used and cleared the middle ear condition in all those who completed the therapy. Interestingly, hearing returned to normal in each child. The doctors remarked that repeated antibiotic use and topical steroid ear drops were likely responsible for the yeast overgrowth of the middle ear.[51]

The identification of microbes in middle ear fluid is useful but fails to provide an answer to one important question. Do these bacteria cause otitis media, or are they merely opportunists taking advantage of a weakened child or hospitable middle ear environment? Without this discussion of childhood susceptibility, there can be no realistic discussion of infection. The problem with the contemporary western concept of infection is that doctors often overlook the question of susceptibility.

Efforts to demonstrate the importance of host susceptibility have, on occasion, taken on dramatic proportion. The great Russian pathol-

	Figure 7			
Types of Bacteria Found in Middle Ear Fluid				
	Percentage			
Bacteria	**1**	**2**	**3**	**4**
S. pneumoniae	29.8	35		33
H. influenzae	20	20.9		23
Streptococcus, g A	8	—		2
B. catarrhalis	11.7	4		
Staph aureus	2	1.6		2
S. pyogenes	3.1	—		
Gram negative enteric bacteria	1	—		
Mixed organisms	2	19.1		7
None or non-pathogenic	29	19.6	42	33

1—Klein, et. al, 1980 (3,583 subjects)[52]
2—Asman, Fireman, 1988 (1,432 subjects)[53]
3—Pelton, et. al, 1980 (122 subjects)[54]
4—Schwartz, et. al, 1978[55]

Differences in the above findings may be due, in part, to the way in which the investigators classified non-pathogenic organisms.

ogist Eli Metschnikoff once drank a solution containing millions of cholera bacteria to prove that a healthy individual would not contract the disease and die. Metchnikoff experienced only mild diarrhea as a result of this experiment. As predicted, he did not contract cholera.

Nutritional status has long been associated with susceptibility to disease. Children suffering from generalized malnutrition are known to suffer from impaired immune function and are at increased risk of succumbing to infections of all types.[56] Overall malnutrition is not even required. Recent studies in the U.S. and Scandinavia have shown that deficiency of only one or two trace elements can render a child more susceptible to infection.[57] Zinc deficiency can cause the thymus gland to shrink substantially, thereby inhibiting cell-mediated immunity.[58] Folic acid is among the most commonly deficient of all nutrients. Lack of this vitamin can lead to reduced resistance to infection.[59] Deficiency of any of the following nutrients has thus far been shown to increase susceptibility to infection: folic acid, pantothenic acid, pyridoxine, riboflavin, vitamin A, vitamin C, vitamin E, copper, iron, magnesium, and zinc.[60]

Lowered immune function, and therefore susceptibility to infection, can be due to genetic factors. Remarkably, it also may be due to the nutritional intake of a parent or grandparent. Evidence for this finding was supplied in a now-famous animal study by Dr. Lucille Hurley, who showed that when a pregnant mother's zinc status is low, the offspring show signs of immune deficiency. This immune insufficiency can persist for up to three generations. The findings are especially significant because the immune problems can often be passed from generation to generation in spite of supplementation with zinc.[61]

Even consumption of sugar can lower immune function by reducing the ability of white blood cells to digest and destroy bacteria. The lowered immune effect can last for five hours or more following the ingestion of sugar.[62] Children with low numbers of intestinal *Lactobacilli* and *Bifidobacteria* are more likely to succumb to infection than are children who harbor optimum levels of these microbes in their intestinal tract.

Environmental factors common today also lower resistance to infection. Cadmium toxicity has been shown to reduce resistance to both bacterial and viral infection. Cadmium is a contaminant of the food, air and water in various areas of the country. It is also found in second-hand cigarette smoke. Lead also inhibits immunity. Lead is found in leaded paint and tap water in older homes, and is a major constituent of house dust in some areas. The adverse effects of both cadmium and lead on children are significant. Not only do these metals cause direct adverse effects on immunity, but they also deplete the body of zinc and calcium, respectively.

Doctors sampled amniotic fluid from 92 pregnant women to determine exposure to seven heavy metals (lead, cadmium, mercury, chromium, cobalt, nickel and silver). A toxic risk score was calculated based on the number and amount of metals present. At age three, children with the highest toxic risk scores were found to have experienced more infections (ear infection, coughs, fevers, sore throat), more allergic illness (asthma, food allergy, insect allergy, noisy breathing, sneezing, rashes and eczema) and more illness in general than those with low scores.[63]

How common is metal toxicity in infants and small children? Dr. Michael Shannon, wrote in *Pediatrics:* "On the basis of these data, it is concluded that lead intoxication in infants is common.... These findings support recommendations that lead screening begin at the age of six months for children with any likelihood of lead exposure." The most common sources of lead in infants was lead-contaminated water used in mixing infant formula, ingested paint chips, and household renovation. In older children paint chip ingestion and household renovation were the most common lead sources.[64]

Unfortunately, many doctors are unaware of the rapidly emerging data that point to nutritional and environmental factors as contributors to infection susceptibility. They continue instead to rely on their arsenal of antibiotics to combat invading organisms that, given the needed raw materials, the child's immune system might defeat alone.

The issue of whether bacteria cause otitis media or act as opportunists cannot be answered fully here. It is likely that under certain conditions, either may be true. There is no doubt that bacteria, viruses, and parasites exact a considerable toll on human health. Every effort should be made to reduce the suffering caused by these microbes. But if the individual child's susceptibility to infection is not considered, repeated infections and continued lowering of resistance may be the result in a significant number of children.

Mechanical Obstruction

Otitis media can occur when the eustachian tube is blocked, or obstructed, by physical or mechanical means. The most common factors associated with mechanical blockage of the eustachian tube are swollen tonsils or adenoids. It was this association that prompted the widespread use of tonsillectomy and adenoidectomy in the early days of treating ear infections. The cause of swollen tonsils or adenoids is not fully understood, but many doctors believe they can be caused or aggravated by allergies. Thus, allergies can lead to the development of one form of mechanical obstruction.

There is another form of mechanical obstruction that further contributes to the development of middle ear problems (and quite possibly the tonsilar and adenoid swelling in some children) called *bio*mechanical obstruction. Biomechanical obstruction refers to blockage that is due to problems involving the structural components surrounding the ear and eustachian tube. These include the bones of the cranium, the TMJ (or jaw joint), and the cervical spine (i.e., the bones of the upper neck).

In other words, abnormal function of the components of the jaw, the skull, and especially the neck can contribute to, and in some cases, cause the development of recurring ear problems.

Biomechanical problems often develop as a result of trauma at birth. Dr. F.R. Ford has pointed out that the spinal column of the infant is very different from that of an adult. He describes the infant vertebrae as a series of elastic cartilages surrounded by **inelastic** connective tissue.[65] This means that the tissue holding the infant's spine together does not lend itself to the same degree of flexibility or elasticity as adult tissue.

In addition, the infant has little or no muscle development. Muscular support of the head and neck is, therefore, non-existent. During birth, extremes of force are often used to pull, prod, or pry the newborn out of the birth canal. According to Dr. Abraham Towbin, of the Department of Neuropathology at Harvard Medical School, "During the final extraction of the fetus, mechanical stress imposed by obstetrical manipulation—even the application of standard orthodox procedures—may prove intolerable to the fetus." He further states that, "During active labor the spinal column, particularly the cervical portion, may be injured as the fetus is compressed and forced down the birth canal."[66]

Tractional forces as high as 67 pounds have been recorded during the delivery of babies. In a study of the tensile strength of the newborn spinal column, it was found that traction of 90 pounds was enough to cause separation and dislocation of the vertebrae, especially in the cervical region. Dr. J.M. Duncan, the principal investigator in this study, comments, "This [amount of tractional force] is probably far from being what most obstetricians would regard as a great force."[67]

These tremendous tractional forces applied during delivery often result in mild to moderate* soft-tissue injury to the components of the infant's spinal column, primarily in the region of the upper neck (which has the greatest range of motion). In many ways, this can be likened to a mild whiplash injury. This microtrauma can occur during prolonged or difficult labor, but is accentuated when forceps, vacuum extraction, or even C-section is used. What may be surprising is that similar trauma can occur even during "normal" delivery.

In 1966, Dr. Viola Frymann examined 1,250 newborns for evidence of mechanical problems resulting from birth. (These births were not even classified as traumatic.) Ten percent of the infants displayed evidence of severe visible trauma, and 78 percent had evidence of articular strains. Therefore, almost 90 percent of all infants demonstrated some degree of biomechanical stress from birth.[68]

Dr. Joan Fallon of New Rochelle, New York, began a pilot study to determine whether birth trauma or fetal malposition played any role in the development of middle ear problems in early infancy. She studied 50 children under the age of six months with otitis media and compared their birth histories with 50 children under

---

*Dr. Abraham Towbin has also found severe spinal cord and brainstem injury that occur as a result of obstetrical trauma even in so-called normal births. This is outside the discussion of this book.

six months who did not develop otitis media. She presented her findings at the 6th Annual Symposium of Otitis Media:

	Otitis Media	Normal
Occiput posterior	11	3
Brow presentation	2	0
C-section	12	7
Breech	5	2
Forceps	2	1
Other trauma	6	0
No trauma or malpresentation	13	37

In essence, she found that children who developed otitis media before six months of age had a much greater frequency of birth trauma or malpresentation. It is also interesting to see the low rate of birth trauma in those who did not develop middle ear problems.

Doctors at Kirksville College of Osteopathic Medicine evaluated 158 children for birth history and evidence of cranial strain patterns. Children with altered head shape at birth (asymmetry) had a 40 percent increase in otitis media. Children with at least three cranial strain patterns at birth had a 75 percent incidence of otitis media.[69]

So, does birth trauma bring about changes that predispose children to middle ear problems? While the issue needs further study with a larger group of children, the work of Drs. Fallon and Degenhardt suggests that there is an association.

If birth (or other) trauma is associated with a higher rate of otitis media, we should find further evidence of spinal, cranial, or TMJ (or jaw joint) problems in these children. Moreover, correction of these problems should lead to an improvement in middle ear symptoms. The evidence for both assertions is growing.

Birth trauma is not the only contributor to biomechanical problems. Children, as any parent has observed, are notoriously inquisitive. Their need for climbing and exploration is matched only by their unending energy. In the course of their explorations, bumps and bruises are sure to come. These occur because of falls off the couch, off the bed, down the stairs, or on the playground. The falls, while usually leaving no outward signs of injury, often result in mild strains of the upper spinal column. It is these minor strains that can lead to problems.

Dr. S. Youniss cites numerous studies suggesting that TMJ disorders are somewhat common in childhood.[70,71] About 20 percent of children aged 6 to 12 experienced either pain, locking or difficulty opening their mouth wide. Half of these children experienced either joint pain, muscle pain, or poor jaw movement.[72]

While these studies were of children over six, it is likely that these problems do not begin abruptly at age six. It is probable that the onset occurs at a much earlier age and is related to factors such as maternal nutrition, infant nutrition, birth trauma, psychological stress and other factors.

If TMJ disorders contribute to the development of otitis media in some children, we would expect treatment of such problems to improve the course of their middle ear problems. Dr. M. Bean noted that by placing crowns on the molars of young children with otitis media the vertical dimension was increased, which led to improved hearing, improvement in middle ear effusion, and decreased need for antibiotic and surgical intervention.[73]

Five young patients with severe overbites and narrow dental arches developed middle ear problems early in life that did not respond to antibiotics or surgery. After correcting the overbite, a dramatic improvement was noted in the middle ear condition of the children. The authors concluded that alteration of the bite (vertical dimension) *may* decrease the incidence of otitis media in young children.[74]

Placing crowns on the molars of small children may not necessarily be the means to solve middle ear problems. These studies suggest, however, that abnormal jaw mechanics may contribute to ear problems in *some* children and that some conservative efforts to restore normal jaw function should be considered.

Functional problems with the bones of the skull may also contribute to middle ear problems (and TMJ problems) in some children. While the skull (cranium) appears to be one solid mass of bone, it is actually comprised of twenty-eight bones, which are separated by joints called sutures. Subtle movements take place at the site of these sutures in a predictable and carefully orchestrated pattern. Restriction in movement has been shown to lead to altered function. The ear canal and tympanic cavity reside within one of the cranial structures called the temporal bone.

For several decades, Dr. John Upledger of Boca Raton, Florida has studied the effects of cranial trauma and abnormal function at the cranial sutures on development of disease. He has published some of the important textbooks on the subject. Upledger has found that in some children with otitis media, cranial therapy restores normal function and improves the middle ear condition.[75]

Manipulation of the cervical spine has also been shown to benefit some children with otitis media. This is especially true when there is a history of birth trauma, obstetrical trauma or trauma in early childhood.

As with any scientific debate, there are critics of this approach. In this case, critics argue that manipulation of the spine has no bearing on improvement of middle ear problems in children. They further suggest that there is no explainable mechanism and that there is a paucity of published data. Although there are many anecdotal accounts and some published case studies of children with middle ear problems who have improved with manipulation, more research is needed to show how this occurs and to what extent this form of treatment will be helpful. The work of Drs. Joan Fallon, Gottfried Gutmann, and others has begun to reveal some very interesting effects of manipulation.

Gottfried Gutmann, M.D., one of Europe's most prominent researchers in the field of physical medicine, describes a case of an 18-month-old boy with early relapsing tonsillitis, frequent enteritis, and therapy-resistant conjunctivitis. The child also suffered from frequent earaches, colds, rhinitis, and sleep problems. The boy's birth had been normal, but he had fallen off the changing table several times.

Examination revealed kyphosis (a reverse curvature) between the second and third cervical vertebrae, and forward and lateral displacement of the first cervical vertebra (C1). After the first specific adjustment of C1, the child improved markedly. Within a short time his ear, nose, and throat problems had ceased.

Dr. Gutmann has reported on the examination and adjustment of more than 1,000 infants and children. His results show that blocked nerve impulses, which result from distortions in the occiput (base of the skull) and the first and second cervical vertebrae, contribute to many clinical conditions, ranging from central motor impairment to lowered resistance to infection. He states that increased susceptibility to infection of the *ear, nose, and throat* is one of the most common consequences of these upper cervical problems.[76,77,78]

Dr. Fallon has been following over 200 cases of otitis media in children. In each case, she has taken tympanogram readings before spinal manipulation and after spinal manipulation. Recall that the tympanogram is a measure of the eardrum that indicates (indirectly) the presence or absence of fluid. A normal tympanogram is represented by a spike-shaped line on the graph. (Figure 7a; Notice that the spiked curve falls within the box.) An abnormal tympanogram

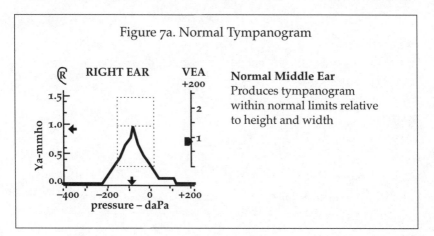

Figure 7a. Normal Tympanogram

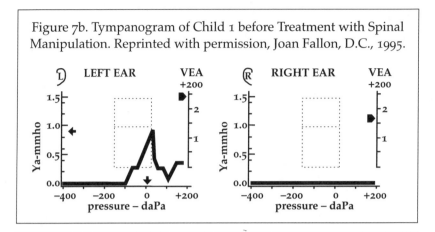

Figure 7b. Tympanogram of Child 1 before Treatment with Spinal Manipulation. Reprinted with permission, Joan Fallon, D.C., 1995.

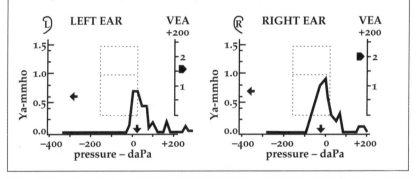

Figure 7c. Tympanogram of Child 1 after Treatment with Spinal Manipulation. Reprinted with permission, Joan Fallon, D.C., 1995.

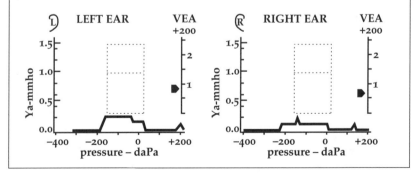

Figure 7d. Tympanogram of Child 2 before Treatment with Spinal Manipulation. Reprinted with permission, Joan Fallon, D.C., 1995.

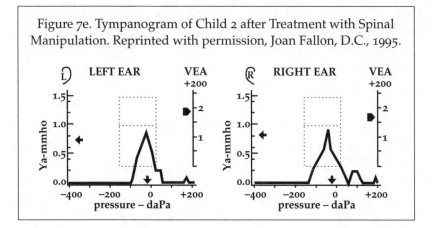

Figure 7e. Tympanogram of Child 2 after Treatment with Spinal Manipulation. Reprinted with permission, Joan Fallon, D.C., 1995.

is represented by a dull curve to a flat line. If your doctor says your child has a "flat" tympanogram, it suggests the presence of middle ear fluid. To date, there is no medication that is directly able to convert a flat tympanogram to a normal tympanogram. This usually occurs only after middle ear fluid has been reduced.

Dr. Fallon has documented many cases in which abnormal tympanograms have been restored to normal tympanograms following spinal manipulation (Figures 7b-e). While the mechanism by which this occurs is not clearly understood, the effect has been observed by numerous doctors in different parts of the United States. Figure 7b represents a child who suffered from recurrent episodes of otitis media since January, 1994. He had received amoxicillin and Septra repeatedly during this period without improvement. The tympanogram shown is flat indicating the presence of middle ear fluid in the right ear (4-10-95). Figure 7c shows the tympanogram (4-18-95) following three treatments using spinal manipulation. (Tympanogram changes were significantly improved within three days of the first treatment). Notice that the curve is a normal spike indicating improvement in eardrum function and reduced middle ear fluid. As of August, 1995, this boy had no further recurrence of middle ear fluid. Figure 7d represents a child suffering from acute otitis media in both ears who had been on amoxicillin for two weeks without improvement. The abnormal tympanogram was taken on

May 17, 1995 immediately before treatment with spinal manipulation. Figure 7e shows a normal tympanogram following spinal manipulation. This child's symptoms of acute otitis media improved immediately along with improvement in the tympanogram. As of January, 1996, there had been no recurrence.

These cases represent only a small number of similar examples of children with chronic middle ear fluid whose tympanograms improved after treatment by spinal manipulation. Do these reports suggest that all children with otitis media would benefit from spinal manipulation? Do they suggest that otitis media is caused, at least in some children, by disordered spinal biomechanics? Does spinal manipulation help these children by improving immune function? Does manipulation affect the neural reflexes of the eustachian tube muscles?

There are many unanswered questions and it is difficult to draw broad conclusions from these findings. However, we should recognize the great potential that exists. Given that many commonly used medical treatments have been shown to have marginal effects on the course of acute and chronic middle ear problems, we should be eager to consider any existing method that shows promise. If this work can be duplicated and indeed shows that spinal and cranial manipulation can normalize tympanograms and improve the middle ear condition, we may be on the threshold of an important breakthrough. We may have available a gentle and safe means to help a substantial number of children.

No one is certain of the extent to which biomechanical problems cause or contribute to otitis media. It will likely take some time and several studies before the role of manipulation in the treatment of otitis media is understood. In the meantime, how does a parent proceed? As with any treatment, parents should consider the potential risks and benefits, and ensure that the health provider has proper training and experience in their field. Otitis media is often a complex disorder that requires an interdisciplinary approach. Parents may wish to consider spinal or cranial manipulation in conjunction with other aspects of care. This is especially true if there is a history of injury or trauma.

These are significant findings. If true, they would suggest that many children who receive antibiotics and tubes do so unnecessarily. Not only do they receive needless therapy with their associated risks, but an important potential contributor to ongoing health problems goes untreated.

Nutrient Insufficiency

Over the past two decades, our understanding of nutrition has expanded rapidly. For instance, we know that a child's intake of dietary fats can either enhance or impair immune function. Intake of the wrong types of fats not only predisposes a child to developing recurrent infections, but to inflammatory conditions as well. Deficiency of certain trace elements and vitamins causes a child's metabolic machinery to go awry, even if essential fats are taken in proper proportion. If all is well regarding the intake of vitamins, minerals, and fats, there are still a host of dietary factors that can upset the balance.

These are important considerations in childhood ear infections. Understanding them can allow you to avoid some things that put your child at risk to ear infections. and to do things that will optimize your child's resistance to disease in general. In this section, we'll explore:

- Types of dietary fats and their sources.
- How fats are made into important substances that affect inflammation and immune function.
- The adverse effects of non-essential fats.
- The role of vitamins and minerals.
- How these factors interact to cause ear infections.
- How aspirin and other antiinflammatory agents can aggravate infection and inflammation.

The information in this section is perhaps the most important tool to developing a better understanding of the role of diet and nutrition not only in regard to ear infections but illness of other types as well. For this reason, I have provided a substantial amount of background information.

Essential Fatty Acids and Dietary Fat

As I discuss the role of dietary fats in middle ear infections, keep in mind that the infant fat requirement is roughly 50 percent of total calories. This is because all developing cells, including those of the nervous system, consist of different types of fats. As a child ages, the fat requirement gradually decreases, eventually reaching about 25 percent of total calories by adulthood. Therefore, the types of fats eaten are especially crucial to an infant or toddler. When a child does not consume fats in the proper ratios, it can spell trouble that will last throughout childhood and even into adulthood.

There are two main types of dietary fats—called **saturated*** fats and **unsaturated*** fats. Saturated fats are those that we typically associate with conditions like heart disease. These fats are solid at room temperature. This is why butter, which is primarily saturated fat, remains solid when left out on the counter top. Your child's body needs certain saturated fats, but can make what it needs. Some saturated fats are useful and some interfere with the body's use of unsaturated essential fats.

Unsaturated fats are liquid at room temperature and are the main constituents of vegetable oils. As with saturated fats, your child's body can make most of what it needs, except linoleic and alpha-linolenic acid. These two are known as essential fatty acids— or EFAs. They are essential because they're necessary for survival and must be obtained through the diet. (Our bodies cannot make

---

*The reason for the designation saturated and unsaturated is that chemically a saturated fat contains only *single* bonds, rendering them more stable, less reactive, and solid at room temperature. Unsaturated fats contain *double* bonds, which make them alterable by heat, light, other molecules, and air. They are therefore less stable, more reactive, and liquid at room temperature.

them.) Essential fatty acids are found in foods such as safflower and flax seed oil.

Besides the two essential fatty acids, there are a variety of non-essential fatty acids in our food. Non-essential fatty acids include those that your child's body can make and those that are artificially created through food processing. Much of the fats found in pastries and doughnuts are non-essential fatty acids created in the deep-frying process.

These artificially created fatty acids can do great harm once inside the body. The problem is that non-essential fatty acids comprise a substantial percentage of most children's diets today.

The Helpful Fatty Acids

There are two main families of essential fatty acids. These are called omega-6 and omega-3 fatty acids.

Omega-6 Fatty Acids. Linoleic acid (LA) is one of the chief EFAs in the omega-6 family. It is found in sunflower, safflower, corn, sesame, flax, soybean, and pumpkin seed. Safflower oil is the highest in LA. **Gamma linolenic acid** (GLA) is found in oil of evening primrose, borage oil, and mother's milk. GLA can be made from LA. Under certain conditions (discussed later), the body cannot convert LA into GLA, in which case GLA must be obtained from the diet. **Arachidonic acid** (AA) is found in animal products such as meat, dairy, and eggs (the only vegetable source is a few select species of seaweed). Breastmilk is also high in arachidonic acid. During infant development, arachidonic acid is necessary for proper brain formation and immune function. Both arachidonic acid and gamma linolenic acid can be synthesized from linoleic acid.

Omega-3 Fatty Acids. The Omega-3 family consists primarily of the essential fatty acid **alpha-linolenic acid** (LNA). It is found in pumpkin seed, flax, soybean, walnut, and in minor amounts in other plants. Flax is the most abundant source, containing 50 to 60 percent of its oil as LNA. LNA is a cold-weather oil found mainly in plants in temperature regions (because of its insulating ability).

Eicosapentaenoic acid (EPA) and **Docosahexaenoic acid** (DHA) are considered cold water marine oils and are found in mackerel, salmon, trout, tuna, cod, and sardines. Like LNA, EPA and DHA have insulating properties. EPA and DHA can be made by the body from LNA and are therefore non-essential. However, under conditions where important enzymes are impaired, LNA does not get converted. In these instances, EPA and DHA become essential and must be obtained from the diet. One reason cod liver oil has been so beneficial over the years is its high EPA and DHA content. Societies which live on diets high in EPA have lower rates of heart and inflammatory diseases.

DHA is increasingly being viewed as a critical component of the brain and nervous system. When present in inadequate amounts early in life (or at any point), nervous system function can suffer significantly.

Changes in Consumption Habits

Food processing practices over the past 100 years have caused the dietary ratio of omega-3 to omega-6 fatty acids to become seriously out of balance for most Americans. While omega-6 intake has remained largely unchanged, omega-3 intake has decreased by nearly 80 percent.[79]

The main reasons for this decrease in omega-3 fatty acid consumption are:

- Omega-3 fatty acids are lost through chemical hydrogenation. Hydrogenation is the process used to turn oil from a liquid to a solid. For example, to convert sunflower oil into sunflower margarine requires hydrogenation.

- 40 percent of omega-3 oils are lost from the increased consumption of southern oils, which are omega-6-rich and omega-3-poor. In the U.S., we consume large amounts of sunflower, safflower, and corn oil—high in omega-6 but low in omega-3.

- Destruction of omega-3 oils occurs when the germ is milled out of northern cereal grains.[80] Essential fatty acids are located primarily in the germ portion of the grains we eat. When grain is milled to make flour, the germ is separated and the endosperm—which is low in EFAs—is sold to consumers. This is one reason that refined (or white) flour products contribute to poor health.

• Fatty acids are easily destroyed by light, heat and air, contributing to an increase of rancid fats in the diet.

Why Your Child's Body Needs Essential Fatty Acids

Essential fatty acids are an important source of energy for your child's body. But when converted into a family of compounds known as prostaglandins, they are among the most potent and vital substances produced in the body. Prostaglandins are hormone-like chemicals that perform an array of functions, ranging from regulating blood clotting to creating inflammation. Many prostaglandins perform dual functions, such as enhancing immunity and regulating hormones. For every prostaglandin that performs one function, there appears to be another that performs the opposite function. This system of checks and balances is in place to ensure that the action of one family of prostaglandins does not get out of control. For example, one prostaglandin family promotes inflammation while another prevents inflammation. If inflammation were prevented entirely, healing would never occur. Yet if inflammation were allowed to proceed unchecked, serious tissue destruction would occur. Likewise, if immunity is stimulated without restraint, it can lead to a disease where the immune system attacks normal body tissue. If immunity is suppressed, we succumb easily to infection.

Prostaglandins are one reason that your child's intake of the proper dietary fatty acids is so important, because only certain types of fatty acids can be made into certain types of prostaglandins. What your child eats is exactly what his cells become. It determines whether he creates inflammation or prevents it, fights disease or gets it.

Some important functions of prostaglandins are listed below.[81]

Figure 8 Sources of Omega-6 and Omega-3 Fatty Acids*				
Omega-6 Oils			Omega-3 Oils	
LA	GLA	AA	LNA	EPA/DHA
Corn Safflower Sunflower Sesame Mother's Milk	Evening Primrose Mother's Milk Borage Pumpkin	Meat Eggs Cow's Milk Butter Mother's Milk	Flax Walnut Soybean Mother's Milk	Salmon Mackerel Mackerel Sardines Trout Mother's Milk

* Most oils contain a mixture of LA, LNA, and other fatty acids. These listings are to show those with the highest content of the fatty acid indicated. Note also that animal products are the only source of AA. LA = linoleic acid; GLA = gamma linolenic acid; AA = arachidonic acid; LNA = alpha linolenic acid; EPA = eicosapentaenoic acid; DHA = docosahexaenoic acid.

- Regulate fever.
- Affect tissue swelling.
- Affect allergies.
- Affect shrinking and swelling of nasal mucous membranes.
- Regulate secretions and their viscosity.
- Cause pain or stop it.
- Regulate smooth muscle (such as those in the ear and those that control the eustachian tube).

How EFAs Are Made into Prostaglandins

There are three main families of prostaglandins, called PG1, PG2, and PG3.* Linoleic acid (LA) is converted into PG1, arachidonic

---

*In this discussion, I refer to the E-series prostaglandins—PG1, etc. However, I have left out the "E" to avoid confounding the reader with excessive technical notation.

acid (AA) into PG2, and alpha-linolenic acid (LNA) into PG3. PG1 tends to control inflammation and enhance immunity. PG2 comprises a family of chemicals that are highly inflammatory and immune-suppressing. PG3 compounds tend to be anti-inflammatory. It is useful to think of PG1 and PG3 as "good guys" and PG2 as "bad guys." (This designation is technically incorrect since all prostaglandins carry out important functions.)

PG1

- blocks allergic response
- prevents inflammation
- improves nerve function
- enhances immune function

PG2

- stimulates allergic response
- promotes inflammation
- suppresses immune function

PG3

- blocks release of PG2 inflammatory precursors
- enhances immune function
- prevents inflammation

Essential fatty acids are converted into prostaglandins through a series of steps that require enzymes and co-factors (see figure 9). The main enzyme is known as d-6-d (delta-6-desaturase). Among the co-factors are vitamins A, B6, C, folic acid, and the trace elements zinc, copper, and magnesium. When these factors are present along with the proper fatty acids, the enzymes work to convert fatty acids into prostaglandins. If the co-factors are not present in sufficient amounts, the enzyme doesn't work, and essential fatty acids are not converted into prostaglandins. Even when the co-factors are present, the enzymes can be prevented from working normally by many factors that are abundant in our childrens' diets today.

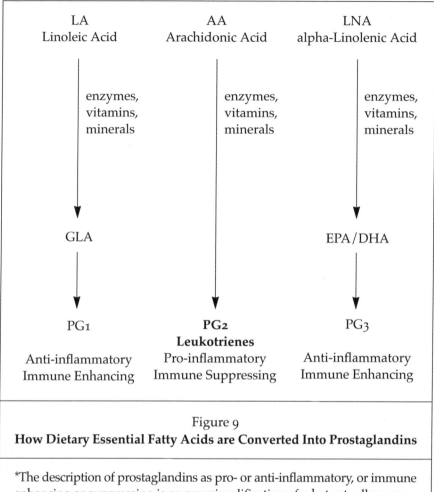

Figure 9
How Dietary Essential Fatty Acids are Converted Into Prostaglandins

*The description of prostaglandins as pro- or anti-inflammatory, or immune enhancing or suppressing is an oversimplification of what actually occurs. However, these designations are useful to show the general way in which these substances affect the body.

Fatty Acids and Breastmilk

One reason breastfeeding is critical to infant and child health is the ratio of essential fatty acids it contains. One important fat found in breastmilk is GLA, or gamma linolenic acid. This is not an essential fatty acid for most adults. However, in infants the enzyme that converts dietary linoleic acid (LA) into GLA is inactive. Breastmilk supplies the needed GLA until the infant's metabolism begins to activate the enzyme on its own. Once this occurs, GLA from the diet is not as crucial.

GLA is necessary for the production of the anti-inflammatory PG1s. If the infant's diet does not contain sufficient amounts of GLA, sufficient PG1 will not be made. If PG1 is not produced in adequate amounts, there is little to oppose the immune-suppressing and inflammation-producing effects of PG2s. Arachidonic acid (AA) is also found in breastmilk. While being a part of the pro-inflammatory system, we cannot think of it as negative for it is a vital component of the developing infant brain. In essence, brain development is impaired if inadequate amounts of AA are present. Breastmilk also contains the omega-3 fatty acids alpha-linolenic acid (LNA), EPA, and DHA.

During pregnancy the mother's fatty acid levels drop significantly, especially the omega-3 fatty acids—specifically DHA. Low levels of essential fatty acids were found to persist in the mother for up to six weeks after birth. This was the end of the study period so it is not clear how long the low levels might have continued. However, since they did not even approach normal at six weeks it is presumed that the effect lasted much longer.

The consequence to the developing child and infant may be significant. It may suggest that even pregnant and lactating mothers need to supplement their diets with additional essential fatty acids, especially the omega-3 variety, to ensure that their own levels remain normal and to ensure that the child not develop inadequacy.

Incidentally, the problem is much worse for children on formula. As of this writing, formula manufacturers do not yet add DHA to formula. They are earnestly studying ways to do so, but adding DHA to formula presents storage problems since the fatty acid is so unstable. This problem will eventually be overcome. In the future, if you use formula, you should attempt to find one that contains both GLA, LNA, and DHA.

Mothers who breastfeed should be aware that the fatty acid content of their diet reflects directly what their breastmilk will contain. If the diet is deficient in omega-3 fatty acids, the breastmilk will be low as well. Worse, if a nursing mother's diet is high in saturated, partially hydrogenated, or trans fats (discussed later), the suckling infant will ingest them and be subjected to all the adverse consequences of exposure to these substances. These non-essential fats show up in mother's milk within 24 hours of the time they were eaten.

The breastmilk of American women tends to be far lower in essential fatty acids than is the breastmilk of women from non-industrialized nations such as Nigeria. Nigerian women consume unprocessed food, which is higher in needed fatty acids and co-factors.[83]

Breastmilk is also a nursing child's only source of zinc, which is essential to proper utilization of fatty acids. During pregnancy and lactation, a mother's zinc requirement increases. It is important that delivery levels of zinc be adequate while breastfeeding to ensure that the baby receives adequate amounts. Recent evidence shows the average nursing mother may only be getting 42 percent of the recommended daily allowance for zinc.[84]

Despite sometimes inadequate amounts of certain nutrients in breastmilk, it remains far superior to formula. No efforts to develop a comparable formula will ever result in a product that matches breastmilk in value to the infant. It is, however, imperative that mothers adopt a diet that is high in nutrient-dense foods and supplement with those nutrients we know to be in short supply.

How Non-Essential Fats Contribute to Illness

Non-essential fatty acids are present naturally in the food we eat. They are also created through food processing. It is those created through food processing that I focus on here. Fatty acids are very sensitive to heat, light, and oxygen. Exposure of oil to heat and air, such as in frying, results in the formation of substances called free radicals.

Free radicals are highly reactive chemical species that can be likened to a lighted match dropped on a dry forest floor. When the match is dropped, tiny twigs and leaves begin to burn. The fire grows and spreads in all directions. Burning embers leap from tree to tree, setting other areas of the forest ablaze in a chain reaction. Eventually large areas of forest are burned. The blaze continues to damage the forest until rainfall occurs or firefighters arrive to spray water on it.

Free radicals released through frying cause chain reactions in the oil molecules, altering their physical shape and chemical usefulness. The resulting chemicals include toxic byproducts about which we know very little. When these chemically altered fats are ingested, they alter the structure of cell membranes, and can trigger chain reactions such as that in the forest. One byproduct created through the cooking and hydrogenation of oil is called the **trans fatty acid**.

Trans fatty acids have a number of adverse effects on the body. They are solid at body temperature, whereas the "good" fatty acids (called cis*) are liquid. They are far more sticky than the "good" fatty acids so they can cause fatty deposits in the blood vessels, liver, and other organs. Normal essential fatty acids are "U" shaped, and are thus recognized by the body's enzymes and incorporated into the design of all body cells. Trans fatty acids are "arrow" shaped and cause serious irregularities in the cell structures. These arrow-shaped fats can slip into the body without being metabolized. They then stick to body tissues rather than being burned as energy.

Trans fatty acids change the permeability of cell membranes. Therefore, things that should get into the cell often don't, and those that shouldn't often do. This latter point is very important because the cell membrane is a vital barrier that protects cells from invading chemicals, bacteria, and viruses.

Trans fats also have a negative impact on the nervous system. Since the nervous system consists primarily of fat tissue, excess

---

*The designation *cis* and *trans* refers to the side of the double bond on which the carbon chains reside. *Cis* literally means "on this side." When the chains are on the same side, the fat molecule is "U" shaped. *Trans* means "across." When the chains are across from one another, the fat molecule is "arrow" shaped. All naturally occurring unsaturated fatty acids are *cis*—this is the form the body must have.

trans fatty acids can cause degeneration of nerves and change their electrical properties. This results in abnormal signals being sent from place to place. Animal studies on this are especially disconcerting. It has been shown that trans fatty acids can be taken up into the brain. When levels of linolenic acid are lower in the diet, the brain appears to take up more trans fatty acids. This is precisely how the American diet is constructed: High trans fatty acids and low omega-3 fatty acids. If the animal studies are confirmed in humans the potential implications are profound.[85]

Among the most damaging effect of trans fatty acids is their ability to cause damage to the existing good fatty acids and drastically alter the production of prostaglandins. (This will be described later in the chapter.)

High levels of trans fats in the diet of children is especially worrisome because once incorporated into the tissues, trans fats are extremely difficult to remove. It takes more than seven weeks to remove half of the trans fats from the heart, and nine days to remove half from the liver.[86] If trans fats continue to be eaten, the residue continues to build and build over time. This gradually changes the composition of the body cells, making them rigid, sticky, and susceptible to damage (such as inflammation and infection). The only presently known way of removing trans fats from the body is to consume omega-3 fatty acids with the needed co-factors (meanwhile reducing the intake of trans fats).

Trans fatty acids comprise from 6 to 12 percent of American's daily fat intake. The most common source is hydrogenated products like margarine and shortening that come from partially hydrogenated vegetable oils. Your child's diet is full of trans fatty acids. Several research studies conducted in the 1980s have shown the trans fatty acid content of common foods to be as high as 60 percent of the total fat with almost no essential fatty acids (the "good" fats) present. For instance, up to 31 percent of the fats in stick margarine are trans fats. (Because of growing concern over trans fatty acids, some margarine companies have begun to manufacture products with lower trans fat content.) Vegetable oil shortenings often contain over 37 percent trans fats. Vegetable salad oils contain up to 13.7 percent. French fries are as high as 37.4 percent Candies, frostings, cakes, and cookies all contain anywhere from 30 to 40 percent of their fats as trans fats. Bakery products such as dough-nuts, some breads, and rolls contain as high as 33.5 percent trans fatty acids.[87,88]

According to research compiled in the book *Fats and Oils,* we consume about 40 grams of margarine and shortening per day (by direct consumption and indirect consumption such as in the prod-ucts mentioned above).[89]

Dr. Maria Enig has studied the trans fatty acid content of foods for some two decades. She has noticed some disturbing trends. When she looked at the trans fat content of a small bag of chips it contained over 25 percent of its fat as trans fatty acids. The total amount of trans fat in one of these bags was up to 4.6 grams, or

Figure 10
The Trans Fatty Acid Content of Common Foods

Food Source	% of Fat as Trans Fatty Acids*
Breads and Rolls	1.8–24
Cakes and Cookies	30–40
Candy and Frostings	38.6
Crackers	20–30
French Fries	37.4
Margarine	
Hard	6–47.8
Soft	6–17
Pastries	33.5
Vegetable Shortening	37.3
Corn Chips	24–30

Journal of the American Oil Chemical Society, Vol. 60, 1983.[90]
Nutrition Reviews, 1984.[91]

*Less than 1 or 2 percent trans fatty acids is ideal.

almost a teaspoon. A serving of french fries fried in vegetable oil contained up to 8.2 grams of trans fatty acids. Deep fried fish filets contained up to 8.0 grams of trans fats.[92]

A single doughnut contained almost 13 g of trans fatty acids. This is disconcerting when one considers USDA data estimating that the average American consumes 63 dozen doughnuts yearly.

Protective Nutrients

Protecting us from the ravages of free radicals and non-essential fats is the **antioxidant defense system**. The anti-oxidant defense system consists of nutrients, including beta-carotene, vitamin C, and vitamin E. Two other powerful anti-oxidants, glutathione and superoxide dismutase, require selenium and riboflavin, and copper, zinc and manganese, respectively. The anti-oxidant defense system can be likened to the rainfall or firefighters described in the above analogy.

When our cells are exposed to free radicals, some local damage occurs. If the anti-oxidant defense system is operating at its peak, the free radicals are "quenched" and produce no more damage. The tissue is repaired and all proceeds well. This is a normal occurrence and goes on constantly within the body. However, if the free radical is not "quenched"—due to a deficiency of one or more of the anti-oxidant nutrients, or an excess of altered fatty acids—a chain reaction begins that can lead to damage throughout the cell. This damage often manifests as inflammation.

Free-radical substances can enter the body from outside sources, including smog, indoor air pollutants, food, water, and radiation. Free radicals are also produced within the body through the normal activity of white blood cells. Our cell membranes are very susceptible to damage by free radicals (and trans fatty acids).

Why Your Child's Important Enzymes May Not Work

I earlier described the enzyme (called delta-6-desaturase) that can easily be prevented from working by either a lack of proper co-factor nutrients or the presence of certain inhibitory compounds in the diet. The presence of these inhibitory compounds can cause both the 1 and 3 prostaglandins to be blocked, leading to the release of only the 2 prostaglandins, or those that are inflammation-producing and immune-suppressing.

The substances that block this enzyme include:[93]

- Saturated fat in excess (typically animal fat, but also includes saturated warm weather oils such as coconut and palm kernel oil).

- Trans fatty acids (described elsewhere in this chapter).

- Oxidizing chemicals (including indoor air pollutants, and constituents of cigarette smoke).

- Aspirin, indomethacin, and other anti-inflammatory drugs.

- Alcohol (cough syrups and other medications). (See chapter 8 for a discussion of FAS.)

- Cortisone (found in many topical creams, nasal sprays, and bronchial inhalers).

- Ionizing radiation (such as X-rays).

- High cholesterol (not a great problem with most children although in some communities up to 50 percent of the children are found to have cholesterol that is considered too high).

- Fasting. (Children usually do not fast, but in cases where the caloric intake is too low, the enzyme may be affected.)

- Refined sugar and flour. (The average American consumes more than 120 pounds of sugar per year.)

- Environmental pollutants (such as lead and cadmium).

- Atopy (an inherited susceptibility to certain diseases such as allergic rhinitis, eczema, and asthma). (More than 70 percent of hyperactive children come from atopic families.)

There are also certain conditions under which the enzymes function poorly. These include:

- Infancy. (The enzyme is not yet active.)

- Diabetes. (In these children, the enzyme is only about 1 percent active.)

- Stress. (Includes children experiencing emotional stress because of problems in the family, at school, day care, or with friends. Under stress, your child's adrenal glands release a stress hormone known as epinephrine, which prevents the enzyme from properly working.)

To function properly, the enzyme requires the presence of certain nutrients in adequate amounts. Included are:

- Magnesium
- Zinc
- Vitamin B6
- Selenium
- Beta-carotene
- Insulin
- Protein
- Vitamin C
- Vitamin B3
- Vitamin A
- Copper

A Trend of Vitamin and Mineral Deficiencies

The diet of the average American child is commonly full of calories and lacking in nutrients. The responsibility for this unfortunate situation lies equally with parents, food manufacturers, advertisers, food growers, and even doctors (because of their general lack of training in nutrition).

Heavy dependence upon chemicals in the growth of food is a substantial contributor to the poor nutrient content of our food. The magnesium content of food is reduced even before processing, due to the use of potassium fertilizers in agriculture.[94] Nutrient levels of food vary greatly from region to region. For instance, the beta-carotene content of carrots may vary many-fold depending upon the area of the country in which the carrots have been grown.

Processing of food adds substantially to lowered nutrient content. The trace element magnesium is often found in short supply in the diet of American children. Magnesium is critical for proper fatty acid metabolism, but high intake of saturated fat increases the body's excretion of magnesium in the urine.[95] Magnesium is located in the germ of most grains. When the grain is processed, the germ is usually discarded, and the endosperm is sold to consumers for use in flour, cereals, cake mixes, and a variety of food products. Processing removes roughly 85 percent of the magnesium from the grain.

Processing of grains also leads to the loss of vitamins B1, B2, B3, B6, E and folic acid. Important trace minerals and essential fatty acids reside in the same portion of the grain as the vitamins. Thus, processing leads to the loss of selenium, zinc, linoleic acid, and alpha-linolenic acid as well. More than 20 nutrients are removed in the processing of flour. Of these, only 7 are replaced through fortification. Improper cooking methods often lead to substantial losses of folic acid, B-vitamins, and vitamin C.

According to Dr. Donald Rudin, anti-nutrients have increased significantly in the diet of Americans. Saturated fat has increased 100 percent, cholesterol 50 percent, refined sugar nearly 1,000 percent, salt nearly 500 percent, and "funny fat" isomers (including trans fatty acids) 1,000 percent.[96]

These changes in eating and food-processing practices have translated into deficiencies in the real world. In *The Selected Minerals in Food Survey* conducted by the FDA from 1982 to 1984, researchers found that daily levels of 11 essential minerals, including calcium, zinc, copper, and magnesium, were less than 80 percent of the RDA for some or all age groups. Among the groups at greatest risk of low intake were children.[97]

Vitamin E is among the most important antioxidant vitamins needed to protect essential fatty acids and cell membranes from damage. It is also vital to regulation of immune function and inflammation. Dr. Adrienne Bendich has reported that a large proportion of U.S. children consume less than two-thirds the recommended daily intake for vitamin E. What's worse, U.S. children were found to have the lowest blood levels of vitamin E of children living in industrialized nations and levels only one-half that of Japanese children. Low levels of vitamin E may play an important role in susceptibility to childhood illness such as otitis media.[98,99]

The Ear Infection Connection

There is direct evidence that deficiency of certain nutrients either increases the susceptibility to or causes otitis media. The reason for this is unclear, but it may be due in part to the need for these nutrients in fatty acid metabolism, which directly affects immune function and inflammation.

Vitamin A deficiency has been shown in animal studies to lead to otitis media. As I described earlier in this chapter, the middle ear is lined with column-shaped cells covered with tiny hairs called cilia. The cilia help to keep the allergens and bacteria from getting into the middle ear by trapping them and waving them down the eustachian tube to be eliminated. It appears that when vitamin A is deficient, the cells lining the middle ear and eustachian tube lose their cilia and become flattened out. When this occurs, the middle ear is not as effectively protected from infection. Vitamin A and beta-carotene (which is two molecules of vitamin A hooked together) are important co-factors in fatty acid conversion to prostaglandins.[100]

Zinc is another nutrient necessary for proper immune function and conversion of fatty acids. Children who are zinc-deficient suffer from atrophy (shrinkage) of the thymus gland.[101] The thymus gland lies directly behind the breastbone (sternum) and is the main source of T-lymphocytes, which are necessary for a child's cell-mediated immunity. Researchers in Sweden report that children who suffer from recurrent upper respiratory and ear infections are more likely to be zinc- (and iron-) deficient than their healthy counterparts.[102]

Several researchers have found that deficiency of various fatty acids in the cells (due to dietary deficiency) leads to abnormal production and release of immune-suppressing and inflammation-producing prostaglandins.[103] These prostaglandins have been shown to contribute to conditions such as rhinitis, asthma, eczema, and allergies.[104] Only recently have we come to realize that the same types of processes might contribute to the development of middle ear infection in children.

When the middle ear fluid of children with otitis media is analyzed, a wide range of inflammatory prostaglandins is typically found. Dr. David P. Skoner and his colleagues studied 102 patients who had persistent middle ear fluid that did not respond to antibiotic therapy. When the middle ear fluid was tested for several inflammatory compounds, Skoner found among them one of the 2-series prostaglandins in substantial amounts. Of these children with inflamed middle ears, only 21 percent had pathogenic bacteria in their middle ear fluid.[105]

At the Division of Otolaryngology-Head and Neck Surgery, at Loma Linda University, Dr. Timothy T.K. Jung conducted an extensive analysis of middle ear fluid for the presence of inflammatory compounds. His work indicates that high concentrations of some of the 2-series prostaglandins (PG2s) and leukotrienes (LTs) are present in the middle ear fluid of children with otitis media.[106]

Some medical researchers are using this information to find new drugs that might block the inflammatory process at various stages. While using anti-inflammatory drugs may be helpful in the short term, it does nothing to correct the underlying problems that set the stage for inflammation. Only by taking a careful look at diet and nutrition (since food provides the fuel for the inflammatory fire) can we hope to understand and correct the imbalances that contribute to otitis media in the immune and inflammatory systems.

This look begins with the fat arachidonic acid. Arachidonic acid is the omega-6 fatty acid found in meat, eggs, and milk. It also can be manufactured from linoleic acid, an omega-6 fatty acid derived from vegetable sources. Arachidonic acid is an important component of the membranes of all body cells. When arachidonic acid is released from the cells, it is quickly converted into a wide array of inflammatory substances—most notably prostaglandins (PGs) and leukotrienes (LTs). This is a normal part of the healing response, since these substances mobilize parts of the body defenses that repair tissue and fight infection. However, if this release of arachidonic acid—with its conversion to PGs and LTs—continues unchecked or is allowed to be triggered with minimal provocation, serious tissue injury can occur.

This is one reason that omega-6 and omega-3 fatty acids must be consumed in proper proportion. Excess arachidonic acid in the diet loads the cells with the fuel for inflammation. If omega-6 linoleic acid is present in excess relative to omega-3 fatty acids, some of the excess is converted into arachidonic acid and stored in the cell membranes. When omega-3 and omega-6 fatty acids are consumed in balanced amounts, 1) production of PG1s, which oppose PG2s, takes place adequately, 2) production of EPA occurs, which blocks the release of arachidonic acid, and 3) PG3 formation occurs, which blocks the action of PG2s and LTs.

Vitamins A and E also prevent the release of arachidonic acid from cells, acting as another buffer against excessive inflammation. Even if arachidonic acid is released, adequate levels of zinc and bioflavonoids can prevent it from being converted excessively into PG2s and LTs.

What are leukotrienes? Leukotrienes (LTs) are made from arachidonic acid. They are 1,000 to 10,000 times more inflammatory than histamine[107] (responsible for the runny nose, itchy eyes, and other symptoms associated with hay fever and allergy) and 1,000 times more inflammatory than the PG2 compounds.[108] Initially, leukocytes (or white blood cells) to accumulate in an infected area.* However, excessive or prolonged secretion of these chemicals can spell disaster. Leukotrienes also produce asthma and hypersensitivity reactions.[109] They are potent inhibitors of immune cells called T-helpers, and potent stimulators of those called T-suppressors. They can, therefore, cause immune alteration when present even in minute quantities.[110] Leukotrienes stimulate secretion of mucus and are found in significant amounts in children with otitis media (especially chronic or mucoid otitis media).[111]

---

*Leukotrienes also perform a variety of other functions.

The events that trigger the release of these compounds in the middle ear are often initiated by bacteria (when present), but can be triggered by free radicals, volatile pollutants, cigarette smoke (which contains both free radicals and volatile pollutants), viruses, trans fatty acids, or mechanical eustachian tube obstruction.*[112]

I described earlier how whatever your child eats (especially in terms of fats) is what his cells become. If the wrong types of fats have been consumed, the cell membranes will be made up of those fats. The cell membrane is the protective wall that surrounds every cell that lines the middle ear, eustachian tube, and the white blood cells that might be called upon to fight infection. When the events that trigger inflammation occur, arachidonic acid is released from the cells. If the proper balance of omega-3 and omega-6 fatty acids have been consumed (along with the supportive nutrients), inflammation usually proceeds only to the point necessary. However, if omega-6 fatty acids are consumed in excess or omega-3 fatty acids consumed in deficiency, the conditions are ripe for continued inflammation and tissue injury.

This may be why so many children continue to have inflammatory middle ear fluid in spite of round after round of antibiotics. In a substantial number of the children who do not respond to antibiotics, the middle ear fluid contains no bacteria.[113] The fluid is, however, filled with inflammatory substances. This suggests either that infection was never present, or that any infection might have long ago been eradicated, leaving the underlying inflammatory changes in its wake. What is likely needed in these children is dietary and nutritional intervention to correct the deteriorating imbalance in the inflammatory system.

---

*It is interesting to note that mechanical eustachian tube obstruction can trigger the release of inflammatory compounds in the middle ear. This may be one reason that spinal manipulation has been useful in managing otitis media in some children (since manipulation can contribute to the reversal of mechanical obstruction).

Why Aspirin and Antiinflammatory Drugs Can Cause Problems

Aspirin and indomethacin have long been used to control fever, relieve pain, and reduce inflammation associated with otitis media. For many years, the reasons for the action of these drugs were not well understood. Today we know that aspirin is a *prostaglandin inhibitor,* meaning that it reduces inflammation by blocking the formation of inflammatory prostaglandins. Unfortunately, there is a substantial trade-off. Aspirin interferes with the enzymes that convert arachidonic acid (AA) into PG2, which on the surface is helpful since PG2 is inflammation-producing. However, aspirin also interferes with the enzymes that convert LA into the anti-inflammatory PG1 and LNA into the anti-inflammatory PG3—this is not good. In other words, anti-inflammatory drugs block the formation of *some* chemicals that promote inflammation, but they also block those that naturally prevent inflammation.

A principal drawback of these drugs is that by blocking the formation of one family of inflammatory substances, the formation of another family of compounds is favored. Members of this family, known as leukotrienes,* are generally more inflammatory than those that aspirin or indomethacin are used to block. Thus, aspirin or indomethacin can favor the release of substances that make inflammation worse. (See chapter 8 for more information and diagrams.)

This has recently been confirmed by the research of Dr. Timothy T.K. Jung, who showed that when drugs such as aspirin are used to treat middle ear infection, the inflammation actually gets worse. Dr. Jung states, "It is conceivable that the free use of aspirin for children with acute otitis media may contribute to the development of mucoid otitis media in these children."[114] Mucoid otitis

---

*Note: Inflammatory HPETEs and related compounds are often produced along with leukotrienes. HPETEs are also found in substantial amounts in inflamed or infected middle ear fluid. They have been left out of the above discussion for reasons of simplicity.

media is a chronic and therapy-resistant form of middle ear disease where the fluid is very thick and sticky.

The adverse effect of anti-inflammatory drugs on the production of highly inflammatory leukotrienes also would explain, in part, the study shared earlier which showed that children with chicken pox recover more slowly when acetaminophen is used.

Cortisone is another drug used by some doctors in the treatment of otitis media (sometimes as nasal spray). Cortisone blocks inflammation by preventing the release of arachidonic acid, thereby preventing both PG2s and LTs from being formed. However, it also blocks the enzymes needed in the formation of the "good" prostaglandins. In addition, cortisone promotes depletion of zinc.[115] Thus, the long-term effect of using cortisone tends toward the suppression of the body's natural inflammation-fighting machinery. According to the new U.S. guidelines on otitis media, use of corticosteroids is not recommended for treatment of otitis media in children of any age.[116]

Based on the available research, it appears that a substantial portion of children suffering from recurrent infections and inflammation may do so because of improper intake of essential fatty acids (and some additional nutrients). Given the ability of aspirin and other anti-inflammatory drugs to *increase* inflammation by further aggravating fatty acid problems, it seems more prudent to restrict the use of these drugs and focus our efforts on correcting the cause of the inflammation.

* * *

As the role of nutrition in both inflammation and immune function becomes more clear, the prospects for therapy based on nutritional and dietary intervention improve, it is likely that many children now using antibiotics and tubes might avoid them with proper nutritional care. Even under circumstances in which antibiotics or tubes are used, careful nutritional management will enhance recovery and may reduce the need for further intervention. The key to this is to demand that your doctor understand the intricacies of nutritional therapy. Children with otitis media should have a thorough assessment of their dietary intake and nutritional status performed.

Solutions to the nutritional problems presented in this section will be discussed in chapters 6, 7, and 8.

In Summary

The evidence presented in this chapter lends strong support to the contention that childhood otitis media is a complex and multifactoral problem. It is rare that all the factors discussed in this chapter are present in a given child. What is not uncommon, however, is to find a dynamic interplay between two or more of these factors. For example, deficiency of fatty acids can predispose a child to allergies. Allergies predispose some children to otitis media. Once the allergic syndrome is set in motion, both nutritional intervention and allergy management must be employed to treat the earaches effectively.

Understanding the causes of otitis media is essential to developing effective treatment. If middle ear fluid is due to factors described above, antibiotics and surgery can only be considered palliative (or symptom-reducing) measures. There will be instances when antibiotics and surgery are required, but it would be prudent for all doctors to recognize the need to address those factors that lead to the development of middle ear fluid and infection.

Chapter 6

Home Care for Earaches

Parents have reported to me that after learning self-care, they are able to cut their visits to the doctor by up to 85 percent.[1]
George Wootan, M.D.

Taking responsibility for home care or choosing to use alternative forms of health care is not a substitute for conventional medical care. As Dr. Richard Moskowitz says, it calls for "a different relationship to the healing process and the health-care system, based on personal choice and direct participation. We still need help when our children get sick, and we need to know that this help is available to us."[2]

It's important that you develop a relationship with a doctor who is at least somewhat supportive of your desire to use alternatives and home care methods. (Most doctors would agree that home care methods are useful if they are not taken to extremes and do not replace common sense.) Also of importance is a family environment where both you and your spouse share a common philosophical belief about how to care for your child. Without this, your desire to use alternatives or home care methods will often be met with confrontation. Therefore, it is important that you discuss ideas and share information.

When to Call the Doctor

Many childhood illnesses can be taken care of at home. But you should always be aware of the general signs that would indicate the need for a doctor. You are often the best judge of your child's condition. The most telling sign of serious illness is your child's behavior. If she looks ill, is behaving unusually, and your instincts tell you to take her in, then follow your instincts. The following guidelines are useful in helping to decide when to take your child to the doctor.

Get Medical Care Immediately:[3]

- If your child shows signs of extreme weakness or loss of consciousness.

- If there is a significant and abrupt change in your child's voice.

- If your child displays or complains of neck stiffness or headache.

- If your child has difficulty breathing or is vomiting.

Get Medical Care Today:

- Anytime a baby has discharge from the ear.

- If an acute earache does not respond to home care within 48 hours.

- If your child experiences a sudden loss of hearing.

- If your child experiences severe ear pain.

- If you see redness on or your child complains of pain around the bony structure behind the ear (known as the mastoid process).

- If fever fails to subside after three days.

- If your infant or toddler continually pokes her finger into the ear canal or tugs at the ear.

See Your Practitioner Soon:

- If a chronic earache has not responded to home care within two weeks.

- If ear discharge has persisted beyond one week.

- If hearing loss has persisted for more than one to two weeks.

Fever: Your Child's Friend, not Foe

Parents in this country tend to be overconcerned about fever in their children. In one survey, more than half of parents erroneously believed that a fever of 104 degrees or less could cause permanent brain damage. Roughly 85 percent gave fever-reducing drugs before temperatures reached 102 degrees, and 68 percent gave their children sponge baths before fever reached 103 degrees.[4, 5]

Contrary to these beliefs, elevated body temperature is an important sign that indicates the immune system is mounting an attack against an infectious agent. When fever is allowed to develop, the body is more efficient at fighting infection. When fever is suppressed, the recovery from illness is slowed.[6] For instance, infected animal pups that are prevented from raising their body temperature have a significantly higher rate of death than those that are allowed to raise their body temperature.[7]

Fever is increasingly being viewed as a controlled response to infection, by which the body raises the "set point" of its thermostat for a specific purpose. According to Matthew J. Kluger, Ph.D., of the Department of Physiology at the University of Michigan Medical School, elevated body temperature results in a modification of the levels of zinc and iron in the bloodstream, which significantly reduces the growth rate of pathogenic bacteria. In addition, fever enhances the bactericidal activity of white blood cells and increase their mobility.[8,9]

A fever is generally considered high only after it rises to 105 degrees. In fact, the body will not allow a fever to rise above 106 degrees unless there is some rare factor present (such as in poisoning or encephalitis) that completely disrupts the body's thermal control mechanism. Fevers of 104 degrees and below are of little concern unless they persist for three or more days. Children commonly experience fluctuations in their normal daily temperatures of almost 2 degrees. The day begins with body temperature has peaked.

This normal rise often gives parents the mistaken belief that a fever is rising. Even when fever rises, it gives no indication of the severity or progression of an illness.

There is a commonly held belief that if a fever rises too high, it can lead to febrile convulsions, and that febrile convulsions predispose a child to developing subsequent seizure disorders. However, convulsions occur in only a small percentage of children with high fever. In one study of 1,706 children who experienced febrile convulsions, there was no evidence of any motor defect and not one single death.[10,11] There appears no evidence that febrile convulsions lead to the development of epilepsy.[12]

The wisdom of routinely giving antibiotics to children with high fever has also been questioned. Writing in the *New England Journal of Medicine,* Dr. David Jaffe reported on a study of 955 children with high fever. Half were given the antibiotic amoxicillin while half were given a placebo. He found virtually no difference in fever outcome between the two groups. Only a few children, who were later found to have bacterial infection, responded to amoxicillin. Dr. Jaffe concluded that antibiotics are "not advisable" for most children with high fever.[13]

Fever-reducing drugs can complicate the healing process with sometimes serious consequences. Aspirin use can lead to the development of Reye's Syndrome, a fatal inflammation of the brain. Since this discovery, doctors no longer recommend aspirin for control of childhood fever. Instead, they recommend acetaminophen. Regarding drugs such as acetaminophen and fever, Dr. Timothy Doran states, ... there is no reason to give it [acetaminophen].[14]

This does not mean that one should never be concerned about fever. But we should always view fever in the context of the general health and appearance of the child. According to one source, fevers usually do not require medical attention except:[15]

- If your child is less than two months old and his temperature exceeds 100 degrees.

- If fever fails to abate after three days or is accompanied by vomiting, respiratory distress, or persistent cough.

- If your child displays listlessness, irritability, or looks seriously ill.

- If your child is making strange twitching movements.

Keep Your Child at Home

There is nothing so disruptive to the healing process as being shuttled out of a comfortable and familiar environment. When a child is ill, she needs peace, quiet, the comforting words of a parent, a gentle touch, and most of all, the knowledge that during this time of discomfort and anxiety, her needs will be fully met. The purely physical needs of child such as providing food, water, medicine, and a change of bedding can be met by almost anyone. Typically a family member (usually a parent or grandparent) is needed to provide the intangibles that are such a large part of the healing response.

For a sick child, create an environment that is free of excessive stimulation. Keep the television and radio off. Dim the lights in the child's room or partially close the shade if the room is too bright. The room should be kept orderly. All toys should be in their place. Tell your child a comforting story. If you need to run errands, don't take your child with you. Wait until your spouse or a friend is available to help. Most of all, show your child extra love and attention, and think about how comforting it was when you, as a child, were cared for by your mother or father.

Avoid sending your sick child to school or day care.* These are environments that are highly stimulating and stressful to a sick child (not to mention the threat of spreading the illness to other children or "picking up something" from another child). A recent "solution" for working parents with sick children is the "day care infirmary"—a day care center staffed by medical personnel (usually nurses). While I can empathize with parents who cannot get

---

*See chapter 7 for day care exclusion guidelines.

off work to care for their sick child, I'm concerned about leaving a large number of moderately ill children together in such a setting.

When Your Child Must Be on Antibiotics

There may be instances when antibiotics will be necessary for your child. Under these circumstances, you must make every effort to minimize the adverse impact of the antibiotic on your child. The first step is to give a bifidus supplement (see section below on intestinal bacteria), one teaspoon, three times per day during the ten-day course of the antibiotic. Doses of bifidus should be given between doses of the antibiotic. In cases of sulfa drug therapy, a two- to three-hour spacing between the bifidus and antibiotic is recommended.[16] Once the antibiotic has been discontinued, continue to give bifidus for one full month.

You also should discuss with your doctor the prospects of your child taking Nystatin with the antibiotic. Nystatin is an antifungal agent that will prevent the overgrowth of intestinal yeast that often accompanies antibiotic therapy. Tell your doctor that you are aware that antibiotics can kill the beneficial bacteria which live in the intestine, and that when this occurs, there is nothing to keep the yeast organisms in check. Convey to him that you realize the need for antibiotics in this situation, but would like to take this additional step for your child. (Incidentally, years ago some antimicrobial preparations contained both antibacterial agents and Nystatin in the same tablet for the reason just mentioned.)

I also recommend that you neither accept nor request an antibiotic prescription over the phone. If your child is sick enough to require an antibiotic, he is sick enough to be seen by a doctor. A doctor cannot discern the state of your child's illness from a telephone call.

What If Your Doctor Recommends Adenoidectomy or Tubes?

Do not accept or reject surgery as a matter of course. If your child has had only a few ear infections and there are no signs of complications, you will want to approach the prospect of surgery with caution. Since ear infections are somewhat seasonal, I would be hesitant to agree to surgery if summer is just around the corner. If your doctor recommends tubes, remember that the likelihood of otorrhea (see chapter 3) is high during summer because of external contamination from swimming.

If your child has had recurrent earaches for some time that have not responded to any therapy, or there are signs of complications, you should consider tubes more realistically. In either case, I recommend that you get a second opinion from a doctor who is in no way associated with your doctor. Ask your friends and family to give you a recommendation, but don't get a referral from your doctor or his staff.

The ultimate decision rests with you. After you have considered all the evidence available to you and consulted with your doctors, you will need to decide what's best for your child. The information I presented in chapter 3 is not an indictment of tubes (or adenoidectomy) and I make no statement about the needs of an individual child. My intent is to present some hazards and complicating features of these procedures so that parents can weigh them against the potential benefits that might be afforded.

Climate Considerations

Fall, winter, and spring are seasons when ear infections are most common—winter being the most likely. An important consideration during these seasons is the relative humidity. In temperate regions such as Minnesota, the outdoor humidity in December falls to around 10 percent and below, while the indoor humidity can plummet to 0 to 5 percent. When the air is this dry, mucous membranes dry out rapidly, causing irritation of the upper respiratory tract, ear, nose, and throat. It will be important to take steps to humidify the air in your child's room. (Adequate fatty acid intake is also needed to maintain lubrication of the cell membranes.)

In contrast, regions such as San Francisco or Seattle become very damp and moist during mid-winter. Dampness also may contribute to upper respiratory and ear problems, but in a different way. If you live in an area like this, it will be important to maintain an area that is dry, warm, and free of excessive humidity. It also will be necessary to protect your child from the elements when going outside.

Emotional Factors

The emotional and physical bodies are not separate entities, but delicately interwoven. Physical distress can manifest emotional changes and emotional distress can manifest physical changes. Whenever illness strikes your child, be aware of emotional and developmental occurrences taking place in his life.

Observe whether your child is having struggles with peers. Is he frustrated trying to master a certain task? Is there a new sibling in the family competing for time and attention? Look at your interaction with your child. In the haste of your schedule, have you tended to rush him? Is your child's environment too restricted? Does your discipline reflect your needs or his? Have you recently divorced or separated? Do you have frequent arguments with your spouse? Have you or your spouse suffered from chronic illness that might be emotionally draining for your child? The list is endless. It is important that you are aware of the way in which events affecting the emotional well-being of your child affect his physical well-being.

I recall a training film designed to show the importance of doctors really getting to know their patients. (This film was based on a study of doctor/patient interaction compared with counselor/patient interaction.) In one segment, a father appears at the doctor's office with his young daughter who had been suffering from recurrent ear infections for six months. The pediatrician walked into the room, asked where the pain was, and proceeded to do an otoscopic exam of the ears. After viewing each ear for about thirty seconds, the doctor concluded that the girl was suffering from otitis media. He promptly prescribed an antibiotic and a decongestant, then left the room.

The study was designed so that a counselor would enter after the doctor had left. In this case, the counselor entered the room and began to ask about their family life. The father broke into tears within moments of beginning to tell how his wife had just died after a prolonged battle with cancer. It had taken a substantial toll on all the family members, especially the daughter. She developed her recurrent health problems while her mother was ill. The sad events of this story illustrate the importance of looking closely at events in our children's lives and listening carefully to not only the overt, but the more subtle signals as well.

A specific example of the relationship of emotion to disease deals with free will. As a child grows and develops emotionally, his will becomes more defined. The will to be an individual, the will to assert his strengths, the will to be free, the will to test limits, and so on, are the birthright of every child. While very powerful, the will of a child is extremely delicate and must be guided and nurtured.

Lending support to the notion that stress affects infection susceptibility in children is two landmark studies. North Carolina-Chapel Hill researchers found that the relative degree of stress brought about by difficult life changes such as death of a grandparent, parental divorce, a move to a new city, birth of a sibling, and so on, was associated with longer duration and severity of infectious illness. In fact, they stated that, "Life change was the strongest single predictor of how long a child stayed ill."[17]

Harvard doctors found that when throat cultures revealed a streptococcal infection, one-half of those under high stress became ill. Of the low-stress individuals with a positive strep culture, only one-fifth actually became ill.[18]

Subsequent studies have shown that psychological factors clearly have an effect on immune function. The response to stress is often dependent upon the child's ability to cope with difficult life circumstances. The key is to listen to your child and look at his or her life during times of illness. Try to foster an environment where your child feels free to express feelings. This appears to be a critical factor in enhancing immune function to prevent illness and to promote recovery during illness.

Children with Down Syndrome

I noted earlier that roughly 60 percent of children with Down syndrome experience otitis media. This is one of the highest risk groups. The structure of the palate and nasopharynx creates an environment that is highly conducive to the development of congestion within the eustachian tube.

Recent evidence suggests that some defects in immune function may be helped by zinc supplementation.[19,20] Selenium supplementation has been shown to improve antibody levels (IgG2 and IgG4) and reduce the occurrence of infection.[21] (Selenium has a narrow margin of safety and should be used under the guidance of a doctor.)

Down syndrome children have an extra copy of chromosome 21, which provides an extra copy of the gene that codes for an enzyme called superoxide dismutase (SOD). SOD activity is elevated by 50 percent in Down syndrome children. Excess SOD activity usually leads to production of free radicals (indirectly from hydrogen peroxide), which can cause tissue damage, inflammation, and altered immune system regulation. To cope with the excess hydrogen peroxide produced by SOD, the body uses glutathione peroxidase, a selenium-dependent antioxidant enzyme. However, this can be used up because of excessive demand. Other antioxidants such as vitamin C, vitamin E, beta-carotene, glutathione and others attempt to compensate, but can be depleted as well.

Because of this understanding, antioxidant therapy has been proposed as an important tool in improving the health of Down syndrome children. Dr. Charles A. Thomas, Jr., director of Pantox Laboratories in San Diego, California has analyzed the blood profiles of 45 children with Down syndrome. He has found that their blood is commonly low in vitamins A, E, and beta-carotene.

Amino acid abnormalities are also common in Down syndrome. Amino acids are the building blocks of proteins, enzymes, neurotransmitters, hormones, and many vital compounds. These children share common traits such as low blood levels of serine, high lysine, high glutamine, and high cysteine. Beyond this, Down syndrome children show a wide variation of high and low amino acids and intermediate compounds. L-carnitine is a non-protein amino acid important in energy production, muscle metabolism and brain metabolism. Trials have shown that acetyl-carnitine may improve brain function in children with Down syndrome. Down syndrome children also present with a complex array of abnormal vitamin, mineral, and co-factor levels.

Dr. J. Alexander Bralley, director of MetaMetrix Medical Laboratory in Norcross, Georgia, has been evaluating nutrient abnormalities in Down syndrome. He has found an emerging pattern of low vitamin B12, folic acid, carnitine, and antioxidants, coupled with abnormal levels of certain amino acids. Low levels of omega-3 fatty acids are also common. Abnormal fatty acid levels are particularly worrisome since it is these fatty acids that form brain architecture and because cognitive problems are so significant in Down syndrome.

In many children, elevated lipid peroxides exist. This reflects the high degree of free-radical stress to which these children are exposed. Moreover, lipid peroxides suggest that vital essential fatty acids are being degraded and destroyed.[23] Collectively, the nutrient abnormalities identified thus far have significant adverse consequences with regard to brain function, energy production, collagen tissue formation, immune function, and development.

It is my opinion that children with Down syndrome have unique biochemical needs. In the past, many doctors have shrugged these off as inevitable consequences of the child's genetic fate, which they presume to have little clinical relevance. Nutrition-minded professionals take a different view. They are of the opinion that many of the altered biochemical findings of Down syndrome can be modified by dietary changes coupled with specific nutrient supplementation. This is in accordance with the emerging view that genetic expression is greatly effected by nutrition and environmental conditions.

The supplementation schedules are based, first, on certain general needs of these children and, second, on biochemical tests of blood and urine that reveal some of the specific metabolic pathways that are altered. These tests must be ordered by a doctor. Tests being used include (but are not limited to):

- Organic acid analysis (urine)

- Fatty acid analysis (red cell or plasma)

- Amino acid analysis (plasma or urine)

- Trace minerals analysis (red cell, hair, other)

- Vitamins (serum, plasma, white blood cells, red blood cells)

- Antioxidant profiles (blood)

- Lipid peroxides (blood)

- Markers of digestion/absorption (stool)

- Lactulose/mannitol intestinal permeability test (See Appendix for the lab results of one Down syndrome child.)

These tests can collectively be somewhat costly. However, when faced with an opportunity to detect and address abnormalities early in life, the potential reward seems well worth the cost.

Dixie Lawrence, executive director of Trisomy 21 Research in Gonzales, Louisiana, has spearheaded an effort to conduct research and build a database on nutritional factors in Down syndrome. Her efforts were spawned by her own Down syndrome child, who experienced dramatic improvement as a result of targeted nutritional intervention. Her story drew national attention. In the week following a segment on national television, her office received 9,000 phone calls. Trisomy 21 Research commonly sends out up to 100 information packets daily. This reflects the large number of families seeking viable means to help their Down syndrome children.

The nutritional protocol devised by the international medical advisory board in collaboration with Trisomy 21 Research is now being used on over 5,000 children in the United States and another 5,000 internationally. Parents have reported consistent reduction of upper respiratory tract infections and ear infections. According to Ms. Lawrence, "These parents report that repeated ear infections not only improve, but in many cases, simply cease to be a problem once the children have been on our program. We have also received reports of improved intelligence, improved motor skills, and altered physical characteristics such as facial features."

Based on my consultation with various clinicians, laboratories, and research groups, I am convinced that a thorough analysis of the child's nutritional and metabolic status can lead to supplementation strategies that greatly benefit many children with Down syndrome. We will never change the fact that these children have an extra 21st chromosome. Our goal should be to optimize their opportunity for good health and attempt to reduce the expression of certain genetic traits. By improving overall health, I believe we can free many of these children from the treadmill of recurrent infections and repeated antibiotics.

Home Care Methods

There are a variety of alternative treatment methods being used successfully to care for otitis media. In all cases, the methods of diagnosis and treatment are complex, requiring the expertise of a trained health practitioner. Home care methods based on the theme of these alternatives can be used with considerable success. Bear in mind that each child is different and not all will respond similarly to home care. One child may experience complete elimination of ear problems using home care methods, while another may notice little improvement.

It is advisable to consult your doctor before making changes in your child's diet or attempting any of the home care methods described below. The alternative methods of treating earaches include:

- Allergy Management.
- Homeopathic Medicine.
- Spinal Manipulation.

- Acupuncture.
- Botanical Medicine.
- Nutrition.

It may at first seem confusing to be presented with so many different approaches. The obvious question is, which approach should I use?

I don't advocate that you use all the home remedies with your child at once. The purpose of showing you this variety of approaches is to give you the opportunity to: 1) choose one that is comfortable to you and suits your personal philosophy, and 2) provide you with options should your child fail to respond to the first home care method you use.

Every child has specific individual needs. The key to helping your child is to individualize the care so it is precisely suited to him. Regardless of which home care methods you choose, you will want to make the necessary dietary changes and follow the prevention strategies that apply to your child's situation.

A rule of thumb is acute earaches respond more quickly, and chronic earaches respond more slowly. If your child has had recurrent infections, multiple courses of antibiotics, or tubes, recovery may be slower. In cases where tubes are used, you will find that healthy children often reject tubes soon after placement. Children who have a weaker constitution will often retain tympanostomy tubes for some time. If your child is among those who has retained the tubes for a long time, it will be important to build up his constitution. This takes time and often involves the help of a professional, although following the guidelines in this book will help immensely.

Allergy Management

Allergists have been around for decades so the treatment of allergy is nothing new. I discuss it as an alternative because conventional allergy management, which consists primarily of scratch testing and allergy shots, has been inadequate in meeting the needs of a large percentage of allergy sufferers. Allergists have also been surprisingly reluctant to acknowledge the existence of food allergy. According to Albert Rowe, M.D., "It is generally agreed that clinical allergy may exist in the absence of positive skin reactions, especially those to the scratch test. This is true primarily in food allergy and to a lesser extent in inhalant allergy."[24]

Shortly after I became aware of the role of food in ear infections, I treated a seven-year-old girl named Melody who suffered from severe exercise-induced asthma, recurrent tonsillitis, recurrent bronchopneumonia, and earaches. Because of the asthma, she was unable to walk a flight of stairs without becoming seriously short of breath and slept sitting up for many months. From age three and a half to age seven, Melody had been under the care of an allergist who routinely prescribed decongestants and antibiotics. The medication helped keep her out of serious distress, but there was little improvement in her condition.

My evaluation suggested that Melody was sensitive to dairy products and wheat. I recommended that her parents withhold these foods for six weeks. With some reluctance Melody's parents agreed to put her on the elimination diet. After one week, she began to improve. Remarkably, she was running and playing with no ill effects. Within two months, Melody was fully recovered, based on not only my evaluation, but that of her allergist as well.

What's interesting about this case is that Melody had gone through a full battery of allergy scratch tests that showed she was allergic to maple trees, dogs, cats, and horses—but no foods. Yet, as it turned out, Melody's recovery was based almost entirely on the removal of offending foods from her diet. The point is that no form of allergy testing is 100 percent accurate. Scratch testing frequently fails to identify allergies that exist. Blood testing is useful, but it fails to identify some allergic children. Elimination-provocation testing (discussed below) is highly valuable, but has drawbacks as well. Because of this, some doctors are beginning to use a combination of tests to verify the presence of allergy. (See chapter 5 for types of allergy testing.)

If your child suffers from recurrent otitis media, you should consider allergy (or hypersensitivity) as a factor. Bear in mind that allergy is not a cause of disease, but the expression of some underlying weakness. Once the weakness is found and corrected, allergies frequently improve.

Ask the following questions to determine if allergy or sensitivity might be involved:

- Did the problems begin in the first six months of life?
- Did the problems start shortly after beginning solid foods?
- Did the problems start shortly after beginning formula?
- Do you or your spouse suffer from allergy or sensitivity?
- Does your child crave certain foods?
- Does the problem subside when traveling away from home?
- Does your child have irregular stools, colic, gas, diarrhea, or constipation?
- Does your child suffer from chronic rhinitis, or stuffy nose?
- Does your child have asthma, recurrent bronchitis, or other upper respiratory problems?
- Does the teacher notice changes in the child's behavior following lunch?
- Does your child develop symptoms following antibiotic therapy?
- Does your child have puffiness, dark circles, or "bags" under the eyes?
- Does your child have occasional difficulty hearing?
- Does your child have difficulty sleeping through the night?
- Does your child wet the bed (nocturnal enuresis) either regularly or on occasion?

- Has your child been on allergy shots at any time in his/her life?

- Does your child suffer from eczema, dry scaly skin, or any other skin condition?

- Is your child overweight or underweight?

- Is your child a "fussy eater?" (Children with food allergies often lose their appetite or taste acuity.)

- Does your child have a horizontal crease on his/her nose or do the so-called "allergic salute?"

If the answer is "yes" to one or more of these questions, there is a chance that your child suffers from allergy or sensitivity to some substance and should be evaluated by a doctor.

Sometimes sensitivity to foods can be determined at home by performing an elimination-provocation test. The object of this test is to remove suspected offending foods from the diet for a period of time (elimination), observe for improvement, and then add the food back to see if the earache or other symptoms return (provocation).

If you are breastfeeding, it's important to examine your diet. First remove any drugs or vitamins from your diet and observe for improvement in your baby. (Never discontinue a doctor-prescribed substance without first consulting your doctor.) Then remove the common offending foods (listed below) and observe for improvement. After five to seven days, if there is no improvement in your child's condition, your diet is probably not at fault. The problem is likely 1) related to your baby's diet (if on solids or some formula), 2) related to an airborne allergy, or 3) unrelated to allergy.

To test an older child, place her on a diet that is free of the common offenders. This includes:

- Dairy products, including milk, butter, cheese, yogurt, cottage cheese, cow's milk formula, and ice cream.

- Wheat, including not only bread and cereal, but anything that contains wheat such as gravies, crackers and cookies.

- Eggs or anything containing eggs.
- Chocolate.
- Citrus, especially oranges and orange juice.
- Corn, or anything containing corn, such as corn flakes.
- Soy. This is especially a problem with infant formula. Dr. William Crook states that 25 percent of infants with milk allergy develop allergy to soy.
- Peanuts, and other nuts. Peanut butter is a great favorite among children and a frequent contributor to childhood health problems.
- Shellfish.
- Sugar.
- Yeast.

In place of these foods, feed your child lamb, rice, squash, carrots, red potatoes, chicken, and applesauce. Observe for improvement in ear symptoms, behavior, runny nose, cough, or any other chronic symptom your child may display. After five days, begin reintroducing the foods one at a time, beginning with those at the top of the list. Dairy products must be avoided for at least three weeks before a determination about sensitivity can be made. Only feed one food per meal, and give the same food for three meals that day. Feeding more than one will confuse the results. When you introduce a food, look for a return of symptoms. Once a child has been off a food for several days, the reaction upon reintroducing can be dramatic.

After you have tested all the foods, you will have an indication of the foods to which your child is sensitive. These foods should be omitted from the diet for several months or until long after the earaches have improved. Remember, earaches are a complex problem. Removing offending foods may lead to striking improvement in some children and no improvement in others. (Note: Children with airborne allergies will often experience a dramatic improvement in their airborne allergies once their food allergies have been addressed.)

A special note should be made about yeast. Many children with recurrent earaches have been on prolonged or multiple courses of antibiotics in their lifetime. Besides having developed food allergies, they are likely to suffer from an infestation of the intestinal yeast/fungus, *Candida albicans* (see chapter 2). This may result in the development of hypersensitivity or allergy to any yeast found in the diet. The diagnosis of a yeast problem is not clearcut and is best made by your doctor. Still, it is useful to know the signs associated with yeast-related problems and the sources of yeast in the diet.

Signs that your child's illness may be yeast-related include:[25]

- History of antibiotics.
- Sensitivity to tobacco smoke, perfumes, paint fumes, other odors.
- Fatigue, sluggishness, lethargy.
- Irritability, hyperactivity, inability to concentrate.
- Fungal infections of the mouth, skin, toe nails, or finger nails.
- Recurring digestive upset, gas, diarrhea.
- Symptoms aggravated by eating.
- Symptoms aggravated from antibiotics.
- Symptoms aggravated when in a moldy area.

Foods that aggravate yeast problems include:[26]

- Refined sugars.
- Anything containing malt (often added to cereals).
- Nuts (especially peanuts and nuts that are not fresh).
- Leftovers (mold grows quickly as foods begin to cool).
- Cheeses.

- Vitamins (especially B-vitamins unless labeled "yeast free").

- Fruit juices (unless freshly prepared).

- Anything with baker's yeast or brewer's yeast listed on the label.

If your child appears to improve while on a diet free of offending foods, the first step is to keep him off the offenders. While important, I believe this is not enough. Allergy and hypersensitivity develop for a reason. Keeping children off certain foods indefinitely is not an acceptable long-term solution (although some children may do well on this type of program). You will want to identify the underlying weaknesses that allow those allergies to develop and correct them. Allergy can be triggered by digestive problems, fatty acid deficiency, trace mineral deficiency, exposure to toxic substances, and numerous other factors. Some of the alternative treatments described in chapter 8 can often reduce the incidence of allergy significantly. For these reasons, the assistance of a health professional will likely be required.

Rotation Diets

A rotation diet refers to the practice of eating certain foods on a schedule. The schedule may consist of eating a food every other day, every five days, every seven days, or some variation. For instance, a child allergic to wheat may have trouble eating wheat every day, but may do well if wheat consumption is restricted to every fifth day. Rotation diets have value in several capacities. First, they can be used in instances where it is unclear which foods are causing problems. Some parents help to reduce illness in their children simply by feeding them on a rotation diet. Second, in cases where a child has multiple food allergies, complete elimination may be difficult and impractical. There also may be concerns about nutritional adequacy. In these instances, adopting a food rotation diet helps reduce her exposure to problem foods, while still providing adequate balance.

Finally, rotation diets can be used when reintroducing an offending food back into the diet. If your child has had recurrent earaches
that have responded well to food allergy management, you will at
some point want to attempt to reintroduce the food(s) back into her
diet—after at least six to nine symptom-free months. (Children
with a history of anaphylaxis related to food should see a doctor
before making any dietary changes.) You first introduce the least
offending food. Once you've determined that it produces no symptoms, add the next offending food. This is done over a period of a
few days. Let's assume you find that all the problem foods now
produce no symptoms. Adding them back on an everyday basis
would be unwise. That might be the quickest way back to trouble.
However, you can add them back on a rotation schedule.

For more information on allergy and childhood illness, see *Is
This Your Child,* by Doris Rapp, M.D.

Homeopathic Medicine

Homeopathy is a comprehensive and effective form of medicine
that works by stimulating the inherent recuperative abilities of the
body. The word homeopathy is derived from the Greek words
homoios meaning "similar" and *pathos*, which means "disease" or
"suffering." Nearly 200 years ago, a German physician named
Samuel Hahnemann observed that any plant, animal, or mineral
substance ingested in excess caused a distinct pattern of symptoms.
Through a series of exhaustive experiments and observations, Dr.
Hahnemann found that these symptom patterns could be cured by
ingesting a minute amount (microdose) of the same substance. This
phenomenon of "like cures like" is what led Hahnemann to describe
the "law of similars" which has become the fundamental pharmacologic principle of homeopathic medicine.

For example, arsenic is a known poison that causes certain types
of fever and digestive disturbance. Homeopathic *Arsenicum* is used
to treat fever and digestive disturbance. Overdose of the plant *Belladonna* results in flushed skin, swollen tonsils, high fever, and
dilated pupils. Homeopathic *Belladonna* is successful at treating
these same symptoms.

We're all familiar with the "law of similars" and the law of micro-doses. Modern allergy practice is loosely based upon it. A child develops hay fever and seeks medical help. His doctor conducts allergy tests and recommends shots that contain minute amounts of the very items to which the child is allergic. However, there are few similarities between allergy shots and homeopathic medicines.

What makes homeopathic medicines different from their some-times toxic counterparts? First, homeopathic medicines begin with a plant, animal, or mineral substance that is diluted sequentially 3 times, 200 times, or even 100,000 times or more. At these dilutions, none of the toxic effects of the original substance remain. It is at this level that homeopathic medicines become powerful healing tools. Another feature that distinguishes homeopathic medicines is the process of potentization through which a remedy must go. At each stage of dilution a homeopathic mixture must be vigor-ously shaken. This causes a form of physical activation. The com-bination of dilution and potentization is what makes homeopathic medicines effective.

The effects of potentized substances have been proven in the laboratory, and in studies with humans and animals. Penicillin, a well-known inhibitor of bacteria, has been shown to inhibit the growth of sensitive bacteria even when present in dilutions of 1:50,000,000 to 1:100,000,000.[27] In 1964, two researchers at the Pas-teur Institute showed that mice could eliminate an endotoxin* when given only 1/10,000 of a microgram of the endotoxin.[28] DDVP, a powerful insecticide, is used in concentrated doses to kill locusts and other insect species. It is also highly toxic to humans and ani-mals. A 1989 report showed that DDVP also exerts insecticidal effects at dilutions as high as 1:10,000,000.[29]

Numerous clinical trials have shown the value of homeopathic medicine in treating disease in humans. In a double-blind study of hay fever sufferers, published in the British medical journal *Lancet*, patients given a 30c homeopathic dilution of 12 grass pollens expe-rienced six times the improvement as those given a placebo. Those

---

*Endotoxins are toxic substances contained within bacterial cells.

under homeopathic care asked for antihistamines only half as often as the placebo group.[30] A recent controlled study showed that doctors obtained good results using homeopathic *Pulsatilla* in the care of children with acute otitis media.[31,32]

A landmark study published by David Taylor Reilly, M.D. and colleagues in 1994, reported that asthmatic children using homeopathic medicine showed improvement after only one week when compared with children taking a placebo. The results were so significant that the authors were forced to conclude that either homeopathic medicine had an effect beyond a shadow of a doubt or that the double-blind, placebo-controlled trial—the basis upon which all modern pharmacology is built—is essentially invalid. They state, "Either answer suggested by the evidence to date—homeopathy works, or the clinical trial does not—is equally challenging to current medical science."[33]

Clinically, homeopaths report exceptional results managing both acute and chronic forms of otitis media. Acute otitis media is more responsive to homeopathic home care. Chronic otitis media often requires the expertise of a trained homeopath. However, acute episodes are common with chronic otitis media, and the acute episodes can often be managed at home with homeopathy. It is my opinion that homeopathic medicine is among the quickest and safest forms of home care available. More importantly, it is one of the most effective.

Potencies

There are two common systems of preparing homeopathic remedies. In one system, one part of the starting material (plant or mineral substance) is diluted to 99 parts liquid. This system is known as the centesimal system—remedies are given the designation "c." The other method uses a dilution of one part medicine to 9 parts liquid—these are designated "x." The number of times a remedy is sequentially diluted in one of these ways is referred to as the dilution. A remedy diluted one part to 99 parts, 6 times, is called a 6c remedy. A remedy diluted one part to 9 parts, 6 times, is called a 6x remedy. For practical purposes 6c and 6x are no different.

Potencies range from 1x (or 1c) to 1,000,000x (or 1,000,000c) and higher.

For home care, it is best to purchase remedies in either the 6th (6c or 6x), 12th (12c or 12x), or 30th (30c or 30x) potency. In general, 30th potencies are deeper and faster acting, but usually require a more accurate remedy selection. Most home care prescribers achieve excellent results using either the 6th or 12th potencies. Proper selection of remedy is more important than the potency chosen.

Dosage

For severe symptoms, the remedy you choose should be given four to six times per day. When symptoms are of a lesser degree, two to four doses daily until symptoms improve are all that is needed. Remedies can be purchased in both liquid and tablet form. Tablets are preferred for children since they are quite palatable. For small children, the tablets should be ground into a powder and given by mouth. The powder also can be mixed with a small amount of water and taken orally.

Remedies are given until there is an improvement in symptoms. Once you notice improvement, the remedy is discontinued. If symptoms resume after a short time, you can give the remedy again. (You may wish to try the next higher potency if this occurs.)

It is not unusual to see dramatic improvement after only one or two doses of a remedy. You can expect most to take longer. If you see no improvement within two or three days, you have probably chosen the wrong remedy. If this occurs, reexamine your child's symptoms and choose another remedy. If, after two or three attempts you're unsuccessful, there are probably other contributing factors.

Healing Crisis

Homeopaths have long recognized a phenomenon known as a healing crisis (also called an aggravation). Sometime soon after the first couple of doses, the child (or adult for that matter) may experience a brief aggravation of symptoms. This is a positive sign (although its absence is not negative) that indicates a deep-acting healing response is occurring. A healing crisis can be differentiated from a true worsening of a child's condition by noting the way in which the changes come about. In a healing crisis, the aggravation of symptoms is usually abrupt and occurs shortly after beginning a remedy. After a brief period of aggravation, the condition begins to improve noticeably. In contrast, when a condition is truly deteriorating, the symptoms may rapidly or slowly get worse, but they continue to decline.

The effects of homeopathic medicines can be profound. In chapter 1, I described the case of four-year-old Tiffany who responded exceptionally well to allergy management. As I related, she had tympanostomy tubes placed in both ears at two and a half years of age. The first tube fell out within seven months of its placement, but the other remained for over 18 months, which greatly concerned the surgeon. Tiffany had been scheduled for surgery for removal of the second tube. However, her parents were reluctant to have her anesthetized again. Two weeks before the surgery date, they asked if I had any suggestions. I recommended Tiffany take homeopathic *Merc dulc* daily for the next week. Within the week, she rejected the second tube. When she arrived at the hospital for her pre-surgical screening, the otolaryngologist told the parents that the tube was no longer in the eardrum and that the eardrum looked "quite good."

Children who don't extrude their tubes within a reasonable period are often constitutionally weak. In Tiffany's case, allergy management helped her earaches considerably, but did not restore her to full strength. The homeopathic medicine improved her constitutional strength sufficiently to reject the tube.

Antagonists

One peculiar aspect of homeopathic medicines is that they can be antidoted by several common substances. This antidoting effect can negate the useful effects of homeopathic medicines on the body. These substances should be avoided when using homeopathic medicines. They include products that contain camphor (some lip balms, Ben Gay, Vick's Vapo-rub, Heet, Campho-Phenique, Noxema), mint or menthol (Hall's cough drops, some toothpastes), and coffee. It is also helpful to avoid substances containing the oils of eucalyptus, rosemary, pennyroyal or other strongly aromatic herbs while taking homeopathic medicines.[34]

Single Remedies

Selecting the proper homeopathic remedy to care for an earache, while not always easy, is rather straightforward. It requires that you observe both the physical and mental signs displayed by your child and match them with the remedy that most closely relates to those signs. It is important not to overlook emotional, mental, or behavioral signs in your child. These are often the most useful in selecting the appropriate remedy.

Following the description of each remedy is a listing of what makes the child's symptoms worse and what makes them better. These are called *modalities* in homeopathic terminology. For instance, the child in need of the remedy *Hepar sulph* is better with warmth, and worse from cold and touch. Modalities are not listed for therapeutic purposes, although there is no doubt that keeping the *Hepar* child warm and avoiding touch will make her more comfortable. Modalities are listed to help guide you to the proper remedy selection. If the child above displays some signs indicating *Hepar sulph*, but is not bothered by touch or cold, chances are that a different remedy is needed.

The remedies most commonly used in home care situations include: *Aconite, Belladonna, Chamomilla, Ferrum phosphoricum, Hepar sulphuricum, Lycopodium, Mercurius, Plantago, Pulsatilla,* and *Silica*. It is important to note that a child need not display all the symptoms of a medicine for that medicine to be effective.

Aconite

This remedy is required when otitis media is caused by exposure to cold wind or a sudden change of temperature. The onset is usually rapid and accompanied by fever. Thirst is almost always present. The external ear is hot, red, painful, and swollen. Anxiety, fear, and restlessness are the most notable mental signs. These children are oversensitive to noise and touch. Unlike the *Belladonna* child, who is delirious and unaware of her surroundings, the *Aconite* child is very alert. The cheeks may be red, hot, flushed, or swollen. On rising, the face may become pale. At times, one cheek may be pale while the other is flushed. This remedy is usually only used in the first 24 hours of an earache that has come on rapidly. Beyond 24 hours, another remedy is usually indicated.

Symptoms are worse: from warmth, a warm room, and at night.

Symptoms are better: in open air.

Belladonna

Belladonna, like *Aconite*, is indicated when an earache comes on suddenly. In fact, *Belladonna* is the most commonly used remedy in the early stages of acute otitis media. The illness is usually associated with hot, red skin, flushed face, glaring eyes, restless sleep, and hypersensitivity of all senses. The throat is hot and dry with swollen tonsils. There is commonly no thirst. The ear, ear canal, and eardrum will often be bright red. Ear pain commonly extends down into the throat. *Belladonna* is associated with high fever that sets in abruptly with little warning. In some cases, there will be few symptoms other than earache and fever. The emotional symptoms are important with *Belladonna*. The child is almost unaware of what is going on around her. The acuteness of her senses may cause her to be agitated and furious, which may lead to outbursts of hitting or biting. These children may have fear of imaginary things, hallucinations and delirium. The pupils are dilated. *Belladonna* should be considered anytime there is intense pain.

Symptoms are worse: from touch, motion, noise, draft, light, odors, and lying on the painful side.

Symptoms are better: from sitting semi-erect.

Chamomilla

This is one of the most commonly used remedies in the care of otitis media. Children in need of *Chamomilla* are irritable and cross. They want something, but when given it are likely to throw it back at you. They are not easily consoled, but may feel better if carried around. They are impatient, and are intolerant of being spoken to, interrupted, or even looked at. If the child is mentally calm, they likely do not need *Chamomilla*. The *Chamomilla* child has bright red cheeks. At times, one cheek may be red while the other is pale. There is acute, stabbing ear pain that may drive the child frantic. Nasal mucus is clear, and discharge from the ear is not typical. The symptoms come on rapidly, although not as rapidly as with *Belladonna*.

Chamomilla is a commonly used remedy for the discomfort associated with teething. If a child is teething and her symptoms match the other symptoms of *Chamomilla* (especially the emotional signs), consider giving *Chamomilla*.

Symptoms are worse: from heat, open air, cold, wind, touch, eating, warmth of the bed, lying down, and at night.

Symptoms are better: from being rocked or carried, warm wet weather, and cold applications.

Ferrum phosphoricum

This is for the child whose earache comes on rapidly, but not as rapidly as with *Belladonna*. The child is feverish but not as severe as with *Belladonna*. The eardrum is red and bulging. *Ferrum phos* is often indicated after exposure to wet weather or when *Belladonna* fails to give relief.

Symptoms are worse: at night and from touch.

Symptoms are better: with cold applications.

Hepar sulphuricum

Hepar is generally not used in the early stages of an earache. It is used when symptoms have progressed and pus has formed in the middle ear. There is frequently a nasal discharge that is at first watery, then becomes thick, yellow, and offensive. There is intense throbbing pain in the ear, accompanied by diminished hearing. These children are irritable and sensitive. Like the *Chamomilla* child, the *Hepar* child is cross and easily angered. They can be provoked to a tantrum with little effort. A hallmark of the *Hepar* child is oversensitivity to touch, cold, and pain. The cold sensitivity may be so great that even a hand or foot exposed from beneath the covers results in aggravation of symptoms.

Symptoms are worse: from dry cold winds, cold foods, touch, pressure, the slightest draft, exertion, or at night.

Symptoms are better: from warmth, extra clothing or covers, humidity, hot applications, and after eating.

Lycopodium

A characteristic of this remedy is symptoms that are on or begin on the right side. There may be a humming and roaring sensation in the ear, with diminished hearing. A thick, yellow, offensive discharge is common. The nose is stopped up. *Lycopodium* is especially indicated in children with digestive complaints such as gas and bloating. These children are thin and weak. They often have cold hands and feet. The *Lycopodium* child is fearful, apprehensive, and afraid to be alone. They are averse to taking on new things. They can be headstrong and scornful when sick. This is a remedy that may be used at any stage of an earache.

Symptoms are worse: from lying on the right side, heat or a warm room, hot air, cold food or drink, eating, and from 4 to 8 p.m.

Symptoms are better: from warm food and drink, being uncovered, motion, cool or open air, and after midnight.

Mercurius

Mercurius is indicated when there is pus formation and is often used in more chronic cases of otitis media. The nasal discharge is yellow-green and offensive (as are all body secretions in these children). There is profuse, offensive perspiration. Lymph nodes are typically swollen. There is great thirst. The skin is almost constantly moist. If the skin is consistently dry, *Mercurius* is not the remedy. Increased salivation, bad breath and puffiness of the tongue are general *Mercurius* symptoms.

The child in need of *Mercurius* is often described as a human "thermometer" because she is acutely sensitive to heat, cold, and most all environmental influences. *Mercurius* children are weak and may tire at the slightest exertion. There is sometimes muscular trembling. These children seem to display a loss of will-power.

Symptoms are worse: from damp, cold, rainy weather, heat,

sweating, motion, exertion, open air, lying on the right side, in a warm bed or warm room, and at night.

Symptoms are better: in moderate temperatures.

Plantago major

Plantago major is needed when ear pain is associated with teething or toothache. The pain often goes from one ear to the other through the head. Intolerance to noise is common. There is a watery, yellowish nasal discharge.

Pulsatilla

This is one of the most frequently used remedies in otitis media and is suitable for almost all types of ear pain. Children needing *Pulsatilla* tend to be gentle, weepy, sensitive, and love to be held. They want attention and are easily consoled by a sympathetic response. *Pulsatilla* children are sometimes described as moody because they can be happy one moment and profoundly sad the next. They often feel sorry for themselves and lament their plight during illness.

Their cheeks are pale. They feel better when in open, fresh air. There is a thick, bland, yellowish-green nasal discharge. The eardrum is swollen and red, with fluid. If the ear is draining, the discharge is usually thick and yellowish-green. The ear is swollen, red, and hot, and there is deep itching in it. The pain often goes through the whole side of the face. There may be a stopped sensation in the ear. A dry or loose cough can be present. Symptoms often come on gradually and frequently follow a cold. The child may be feverish, but show a surprising absence of thirst.

Symptoms are worse: from heat, lying down, exertion, after eating, toward evening, and in a warm room.

Symptoms are better: from motion, cold applications, cold food and drink, and in open air.

Silica

Children in need of *Silica* are likely to experience discharge from the ear. They are sensitive and anxious. *Silica* is often indicated when a cold or bronchial condition is long-standing or slow to respond. Symptoms are severe. There is often roaring in the ears, and the child is sensitive to noise. The *Silica* child is cold, chilly, and wants plenty of warm clothing. He hates drafts, and his hands and feet are icy cold. There is offensive sweat on the hands, feet, and armpits. *Silica* is the remedy most often indicated when there is pain behind the ear on the mastoid process. (See also *Hepar sulph*.)

Mentally these children are yielding, faint-hearted, and anxious. They are nervous, excitable, and sensitive, but can be obstinate. *Silica* children tend to be weak and easily exhausted.

Symptoms are worse: from cold, open air, winter, damp weather, cold food or drink, lying on the painful side, eating, and in morning.

Symptoms are better: from warmth.

It is not always easy to decide which homeopathic medicine your child might need. Often the choice can be narrowed down to two or three medicines, but the final selection can be difficult. To make this process easier, a series of flow charts has been designed by Dr. Stephen Messer. These charts can be found in chapter 8 under Homeopathic Medicine. The figures labeled Otitis Media Without Effusion and Acute Otitis Media are those most likely to be useful in home care. Recognize that proper use of these charts depends upon making a specific diagnosis of the middle ear condition.

Ear Drops

Ear drops are discussed in the section on botanical medicine, but one excellent homeopathic eardrop formula deserves mention here. **Traumeel** is a patent formula made by Biological Homeopathic Industries. David Riley, M.D., reports that Traumeel applied topically can provide substantial relief when ear pain strikes. It can be purchased in liquid form. To apply this formula, warm several drops on a teaspoon, then place 3 drops in each ear and cover with cotton. (This is not for use in an ear where you see drainage.)

Traumeel consists of:*

---

*The "D" designation is equivalent to the "x" discussed above.

Arnica D2
Hamamelis D2
Belladonna D4
Hepar sulfuris D5
Chamomilla D3
Bellis perennis D2
Echinacea purpurea D2
Calendula D2
Millefolium D3
Aconitum D3
Mercuris solubilis Hahnemanni D8
Symphytum D3
Echinacea angustifolia D2
Hypericum D2

Colds and Nasal Congestion

Homeopathic medicine is very effective at treating the symptoms of colds, sinus, and nasal congestion that often precede otitis media. If your child is prone to earaches, any cold or sinus problem should be managed homeopathically. The appropriate remedies are discussed in chapter 7.

For more information on homeopathic medicine, I suggest you read the books *Homeopathy: Medicine for the Twenty-first Century,* by Dana Ullman, M.P.H., and *Everybody's Guide to Homeopathic Medicines,* by Stephen Cummings, M.D., and Dana Ullman, M.P.H.

Rather than simply purchasing individual remedies, I recommend that parents purchase a homeopathic remedy kit. Kits come in all sizes, ranging from those that contain 10 remedies all the way up to 50. Having a variety of remedies at your disposal will allow you to administer home care for many common childhood complaints including colic, upset stomach, colds, bumps, bruises, and more.

To order books and remedies, see the resource section of this book.

Spinal Manipulation

The use of manipulation of the vertebrae and other joints of the body has been a part of medical systems throughout recorded history. The Chinese have used manipulation for more than two thousand years as an integral part of their medical system. During the time of Hippocrates, manipulation of the vertebrae was used to treat a variety of disorders, especially those of a musculoskeletal origin. Manipulation of the vertebrae (and other joints) has seen a rapid rebirth in contemporary Western medicine through the practice of chiropractic and osteopathy. The body of evidence of the therapeutic value of manipulation is growing steadily.

When biomechanical problems of the upper spine contribute to otitis media, correction of these problems becomes an integral part of treatment. Dr. Gottfried Gutmann makes three important points on biomechanical problems, manipulation, and recurrent infections. He concludes that: 1) blocked nerve impulses at the atlas [first cervical vertebrae] contribute to lower resistance to infections of the ear, nose and throat, 2) chiropractic and radiological examinations are "of decisive importance" for diagnosis of the syndrome, and 3) "chiropractic can often bring about amazingly successful results, because the therapy is a causal one."[35,36]

Manipulation is discussed here not because it is a method of home care, but to show its place in the overall scheme of how otitis media must be viewed from a treatment perspective. In cases of biomechanical problems that require manipulation, a doctor of chiropractic or osteopathy must be consulted. See chapter 8 for a more detailed discussion of manipulation.

Acupressure

The practice of Chinese medicine traditionally includes diet, exercise, manipulation, massage, meditation, bone-setting, herbs and acupuncture. The term acupuncture describes one of many methods of stimulating various locations on the body known as acupoints. Acupressure is another common means of stimulating these points.

Over the years, the Chinese have discovered that specific acupoints have specific functions. The stimulation of these points causes predictable changes to occur throughout the body.

For example, the point Large Intestine 4 is said to eliminate pathogenic wind from the head and face. Crudely translated, pathogenic wind refers to viral influences. (The Chinese lacked knowledge of viruses as we know them today, but their clinical descriptions are profoundly accurate.) In practice, Large Intestine 4 (LI-4) has a significant effect on symptoms of headache, toothache, sore throat, fever, earache, and the common cold. Thus, the point LI-4 would be stimulated in certain types of earaches.

The point San Jiao 5 (SJ-5, or TH-5) is known to expel wind (thus having an influence on what we would call viral syndromes) and regulate the San Jiao channel. The San Jiao channel refers to a meridian, or pathway, through which energy travels. The San Jiao channel circles the ear and sends a branch through the ear. Regulation of this channel is important in correcting the problems that exist during an ear infection. In actual practice, treating San Jiao 5 can have remarkable effects on the progress of otitis media. I've observed acute inflammatory middle ear problems resolve fully in just 24 hours using this and one other point.

What if an earache occurs with high fever, signs of heat, and inflammation that does not subside? In Chinese medicine this is called pathogenic wind-heat. This description, while foreign to Westerners, tells the acupuncturist that points must be used that will dissipate or clear this wind-heat. One point which serves this purpose is called Du-14. Clinically, this point is used in febrile illnesses, the common cold, cough, asthma, and earache. Du-14 is used with other pertinent acupoints to correct the underlying syndrome that has manifested as middle ear inflammation. In the Chinese system of medicine, there are points that cover the whole range of therapeutic application. This makes Chinese medicine an extremely useful and versatile system of healing.

In Chinese medicine, illness is not viewed as a cause and effect phenomenon. The Chinese view illness as an expression of patterns of disharmony. The acupuncturist makes his diagnosis based upon a careful physical examination of the patient. Questions about the child's behavior, habits, and symptomatology are asked. This information is used to identify the pattern involved. Once the pattern has been identified, the acupuncturist selects the points (usually only 2–4 points with children) that would be most successful in correcting the underlying disharmony. The points are then stimulated for a brief period using needles, pressure, or any number of other methods employed today. It is important to note that the results of acupuncture are enhanced by the concurrent use of botanical medicine.

Acupressure for Earaches

You obviously won't be doing acupuncture at home, but you can use acupressure, which is often very effective at alleviating the symptoms of earache. Stimulating acupoints with pressure is useful because it can influence lymph drainage, reduce pain, and sometimes encourage removal of fluid from the middle ear.

To treat the acupoints, have your child lie down comfortably on the bed. First, locate all of the points you will be treating. (See figure 11.) You'll notice that some points are near the ear while others are as far away as the foot. In this treatment, you begin with the point furthest from the ear. Once you have stimulated it, you go to the next closest, and so on.

Stimulation of the point is achieved by placing your thumb over it and placing slight to moderate pressure in a gentle massaging motion. Continue this for one minute. If the pressure you are using causes pain, ease up a little. As you get to the points closest to the ear, you may find they are so tender that your child will not let you touch them. If this is the case, avoid these points.

The points used in the home care of earaches, in order of first treated to last are:

1. GB-41
2. KI-7
3. KI-3
4. LI-4
5. TH-5
6. GB-20
7. TH-17 (gently)
8. GB-2

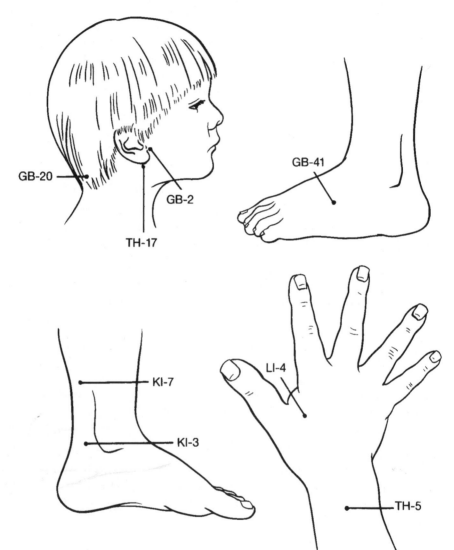

Figure 11
Accupoints Used in Otitis Media

This acupressure treatment can be done two to three times per day.

Clearing Lymphatic Congestion

Another useful method that can be employed at home when a case of otitis media occurs is the "Lymphatic Flush," used to enhance the function of the tonsils and adenoids.

The tonsils and adenoids are part of the lymphatic system. Connecting these and other lymph structures, including lymph nodes, is a large network of lymphatic vessels. It is the job of the lymphatic vessels to transport waste products throughout the body to be eliminated. They also serve as a pathway for the movement of white blood cells to the site of infection.

At times, flow through the lymphatic vessels of the head and neck is reduced due to swelling, inflammation, mechanical obstruction, infection, allergy, and so on. If the lymphatic vessels don't drain, the tonsils and adenoids cannot eliminate waste products and thus become more swollen. This leads to obstruction of the eustachian tube, preventing normal drainage. Impaired drainage results in fluid accumulation in the middle ear and aggravation of ear pain.

The lymphatic flush technique can be done at home to enhance drainage and improve the environment around the eustachian tube. This often greatly enhances the healing of the middle ear. I've recommended this to parents for years. The results are exceptional.

The Lymphatic Flush (see figure 12)

1. Have your child lie down on his back, with his head slightly elevated.

2. Apply a generous helping of unscented hand lotion to your hands. Make sure that your hands and the lotion are warm.

3. Gently rub the lotion up and down the front and sides of your child's neck. This will spread the lotion and also get your child accustomed to your touch. Remember, he is in pain so proceed slowly.

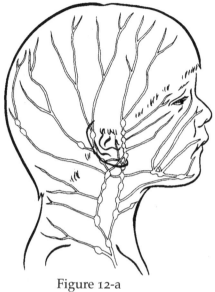

Figure 12-a
Lymph Nodes of the Head and Neck

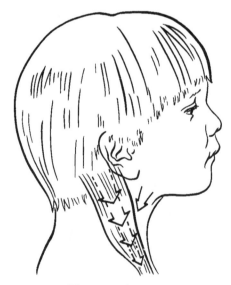

Figure 12-b
Lymphatic Flush Technique

4. The area you're treating lies along the large muscle which is located on the front and side of the neck (called the sternocleidomastoid). Using a broad hand contact, and beginning about one inch up from the collarbone on each side (the dimensions will vary depending upon the age and size of the child), stroke your hand downward in the direction of the collarbone. Use moderate pressure and repeat five or six times.

5. Place your hands two inches up from the collarbone and stroke downward five or six times.

6. Next, place your hands one inch higher than the previous time and stroke downward five or six times.

7. Repeat this until your hands are up at the tonsils. At this point, you will be making long strokes from the tonsils downward.

The purpose of this exercise is to encourage fluid to drain away from the tonsils, thus reducing the amount of congestion in that area. You begin at the bottom because it is necessary to clear an area of stagnant lymph fluid. Once the lower lymph vessels are open, it will be easier to move the above fluid downward. This technique can provide substantial relief to an ailing child.

Spinal Massage

The spinal massage is done by having your child lie down on the bed on his belly. It can be done with your child's shirt on or off, depending on which is more comfortable to him. I prefer to stimulate the bare skin. If you do this, use unscented lotion, and make sure your hands and the room are warm enough.

With your child on his belly, begin in the small of the back and massage along both sides of the spine, working your way upward as you go. Work slowly and gently, spending about 30 seconds at each level. Continue until you reach the base of the skull. The entire exercise should take roughly ten minutes.

There are three main reasons for doing this procedure. First,

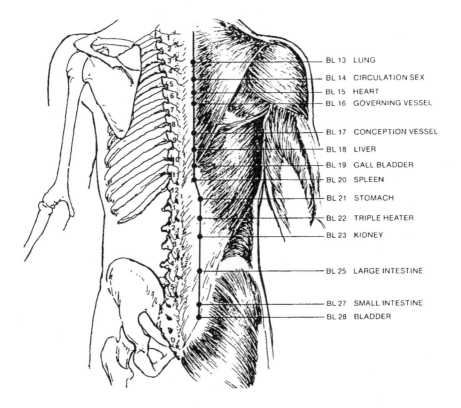

Figure 13
Association Points of Acupuncture

treatment of this area stimulates drainage of some of the lymphatic vessels affecting the lungs. Second, the autonomic nervous system can be influenced. (This part of the nervous system controls automatic functions such as secretion of mucus.) And third, the acupuncture association points are stimulated. (See figure 13.) All along the spinal column lie acupuncture points that associate with each major organ system. General stimulation of these points can enhance the integrated functions of the body during illness.

Children love to be massaged. You will be amazed at how much this can improve your child's well-being and enhance his recovery.

Acupressure for Colds and Nasal Congestion

The longer the nasal cavity remains congested, the greater the likelihood of congestion developing in the middle ear. A simple acupressure treatment can often aid in reducing nasal congestion. (Obviously if other factors exist, you will have to identify these as well.)

1. Have your child lie down on his back with his head slightly elevated. You should be seated at his head.

2. Using the pads of your fingers, gently massage the points listed in figure 14.

3. Spend about 45 seconds treating each point. The entire treatment should take about 7 minutes.

The points used in the treatment of colds and nasal congestion include:

1. DU-16
2. DU-20
3. BL-12
4. GB-20
5. LI-20
6. BL-4
7. LU-7

Botanical Medicine

The use of plants to treat disease is perhaps the oldest form of medicine known. Today, both botanical medicine and allopathic medicine depend heavily upon the same plants used centuries ago. nearly 70 percent of today's patent drugs are manufactured using knowledge of plant substances, and 25 percent have substances extracted directly from plants. For example, the drug Ephedra is used widely in the west to treat respiratory conditions. This is derived from the Chinese plant known as Ma Huang, or *Ephedra sinica*. The use of Ma Huang to treat respiratory conditions was documented in Chinese medical literature centuries ago.

For hundreds of years herbalists treated colds, inflammation, and pain by having patients chew on the bark of black willow, or

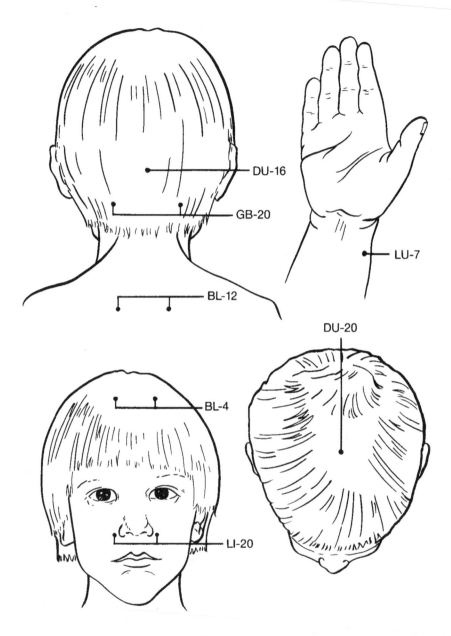

Figure 14
Acupoints for Colds and Nasal Congestion

meadowsweet. Today we take it in the form more commonly known as aspirin, the name of which is derived from the old botanical name of meadowsweet, Spirea.[37]

The clinical results obtained in the skilled practice of botanical medicine worldwide are impressive. Clinical and laboratory studies in the West continue to elucidate the specific actions of plant substances. For instance, St. John's Wort *(Hypericum triquetrifolium)* has been shown to interfere with viral infection and replication.[38] Constituents found in the *shitake* mushroom *(Lentinus edodes)* affect viruses indirectly by enhancing T and B lymphocyte function and stimulating natural killer cells. This plant also has anti-tumor activity.[39]

The common milk thistle *(Silybum marianum)* contains, as its chief active ingredient, a compound called silymarin, which is reputed to be one of the most potent liver-protecting substances known. Silymarins are powerful antioxidants. This compound stimulates the production of new liver cells to replace damaged cells. Studies in Finland, Russia, and Europe have shown this healing effect to occur in people with sustained liver damaged due to diabetes, alcohol, drugs, environmental toxins, and viruses.[40]

Given the rich history of botanical medicine and the emerging scientific confirmation of its value, it is no surprise that botanical medicine has a role to play in the management of childhood otitis media. Recently, Ikeda and Takasaka reported a study using Kampo medicine to treat secretory otitis media. Kampo medicine, or *Sairei-to,** as it's called in Japan, consists of eight different herbs. This investigation was based on evidence that Kampo medicine is effective in resolving conditions that exhibit inflammatory and immunological reactions. An advantage of using Kampo medicine is that it causes few adverse effects even in long-term treatment—a desirable feature where children are concerned. At the completion of this four-week trial, the authors concluded that "Kampo medicine may resolve the inflammation and immune response associated

---

*Sairei-to consists of the herbs *Bupleurum falcatum, Alisma orientale, Pinellia ternata, Scutellaria baicalensis, Zizyphus jujuba, Panax ginseng, Cinnamomum cassia,* and *Zingiber offinale.*

with secretory otitis media."[41]

While botanical medicine can be helpful in managing otitis media, prescribing herbal combinations is a complex process. There are numerous different syndromes in otitis media, each of which requires different herbal formulas. Thus, for home care purposes, I've listed only those that 1) are used as ear drops to relieve pain, 2) build energy in constitutionally weak children, and 3) act as general immune stimulants.

Ear Drops

Ear drops are not generally known to cure earaches, but they can provide what most parents and children are after—relief of symptoms. The most effective herbs used as drops include:

- *Plantago major* tincture.
- *Pennywort* tincture.
- *Mullein* oil.
- *Chamomile* infusion.
- *Olive* oil.
- The Three Yellows (see chapter 8).

It's only necessary to use one of the above at any given time. I've listed several because you may find that one does not work for your child. In such a case, choose another on the list. I've found *Plantago major* to be very effective, especially when the earaches are associated with teething problems. Martha Benedict, an acupuncturist in Santa Cruz, California, claims exceptional results using the three yellows.[42]

The herb solution should be heated slightly by placing a few drops on a spoon and warming it for a few seconds with a match from underneath. Using a dropper, which is usually provided with the herbal mixture, withdraw the herb from the spoon and test a drop on the inside of your wrist to make sure it is not too warm. Next, place three drops in the affected ear and cover with a piece of cotton. The application should be repeated three times per day during the course of the earache. You may wish to use the same piece of cotton for a day or two, since it will be saturated and less likely to absorb the herb the next time you use it in the ear. Eardrops should not be used when there is fluid draining out of the middle ear.

Most of the above herbs are available at health food stores or can be ordered from the companies listed in the resource section.

Herbal Teas

Herbal teas can be used to reduce mucous congestion and build energy in a weakened or sick child.

For children with excessive mucus production, you can make a tea that consists of water, one-eighth teaspoon of raw honey, a few drops of brandy, and fresh ground ginger root, cinnamon, or cayenne.

Nose Drops

Clearing the nasal passages can sometimes help speed recovery of the middle ear. In addition, clear nasal passages allow the child to breathe more easily, which goes a long way toward ensuring a much-needed night's sleep for both you and your child.

One type of nose drop that occasionally proves helpful is a simple saltwater solution. This can be made by placing one teaspoon of table salt in a quart of warm water.

A nose drop that works exceptionally well is a mixture of fennelated Irish moss. Place one drop in the child's right nostril, then one in the left. Repeat until four drops have been placed in each nostril. At the time the first drop is placed, your child may notice a slight stinging sensation that quickly goes away once the second drop is applied and the Irish moss begins to do its work. The nose drops should be used four times a day during the active phase of an earache.

General Immune Stimulants

The most common botanical used in the West to enhance immune function is *Echinacea*. There have been more than 200 laboratory and clinical studies on the physiological effects of this herb. *Echinacea* has been shown to be anti-viral, anti-bacterial, and anti-fungal. Its use as a general immune tonic is widely known. Up to about 1930 and prior to the discovery of sulfa drugs, *Echinacea* was used regularly by physicians throughout the United States.[43]

Echinacea is usually purchased in tincture form. Five drops in a small glass of water can be given orally three times daily to a child over two. Under two years, give three drops three times daily.

Nutrition

Nutritional home care for earaches is a somewhat new area, and much remains to be learned. Still, there are certain fundamental approaches that can be used, based upon what we know about nutrition and inflammation, and nutrition and immune function.

Listed below are some nutrients that are useful in times of earache. I do not advise that all the items listed below be given in separate tablets. The list is provided as a guideline to suggest the nutrients that should be included in a multivitamin. Supplements such as evening primrose oil, flax oil, bifidus, acidophilus, and proanthocyanadins are given separately.

A child who suffers from either acute or chronic earaches can be given:

ages 1–3	ages 4 and up
500 mg vitamin C	1,000 to 1,500 mg vitamin C
25–50 IU vitamin E	50 IU vitamin E
1,000 IU vitamin A	1,000 IU vitamin A
5,000 IU beta-carotene	5,000 IU beta-carotene
50 mg magnesium	75 mg magnesium
5–10 mg zinc*	10 mg zinc*
10mg coenzyme Q10	20 mg coenzyme Q10
1 children's B-complex	1 children's B-complex
1 tsp flax oil	1.5 tsp flax oil
1 perle borage oil	2 perle borage oil
25 mg proanthocyanadin	25–50 mg proanthocyanadin
1 tsp Bifidus/acidophilus	1–2 tsp. Bifidus/acidophilus

In addition to the above program, you may wish to add about 50 mg of DHA, or 1 perle/day.** (See appendix for sources.)

Zinc and vitamin C can often be given together in a lozenge that is now available commercially. A child who chews these lozenges should have his teeth brushed afterward since ascorbic acid can be harmful to the enamel after prolonged contact with the teeth. Additional beta-carotene can be obtained by eating more orange and yellow vegetables such as carrots and squash. Vitamin A has a separate but important immune potentiating effect. Omega-3 fatty acids can be obtained from flax oil, fish oil, or from the special DHA-containing product mentioned above.

Bifidobacteria are not found in any food products and therefore must be purchased as a supplement (see discussion of acidophilus and bifidus). During an earache, avoid feeding your child sugar in any form—this includes fruit juice. A study at Loma Linda School of Medicine showed that fructose, sucrose, honey, or orange juice all significantly decreased the capacity of neutrophils (a white blood cell) to engulf bacteria. Children who are ill often don't feel like eating, and it's a good idea to follow their lead. During any type of infection or inflammation, the need for liquids increases so be sure to provide plenty of fluids.

A plant substance that has received widespread attention is called Pycnogenol. Pycnogenol is a trade name for a complex of flavonoid compounds derived from the maritime pine. The flavones, flavonones, and flavonols are referred to collectively as proanthocyanadins. Grape seed is another very potent source of these compounds. Clinicians in the United States, Europe, and elsewhere are finding that the substantial antiinflammatory properties of proantho-

---

*Make sure the supplement contains about 3 micrograms of copper to balance with zinc. Do not give more zinc in hopes that more will stimulate the immune system better. Excess zinc inhibits immune function.

**Do not give perles to children under four or five. Break the perles open, and express the oil. Give the oil to your child by mouth or add it to juice, formula, or food. The proper dosage for children is one perle per year of age per day, up to six perles per day.

cyanadins are of great value in many disorders. Various doctors have reported their success in using proanthocyanadins as a component of earache treatment.

Iron is necessary for fighting infection. Yet, excess iron can cause a variety of problems including immune suppression. I don't recommend that anyone take additional iron unless directed by their doctor. Doctors prescribing iron to patients should have good clinical or laboratory evidence of the need for iron before prescribing it. The best way for a child to obtain iron is from food. Nuts, blackstrap molasses, and dark turkey meat are good sources of iron. Iron absorption is enhanced when iron is taken with vitamin C-containing foods.

Since fatty acid imbalance plays such a large role in illness, it is important that you recognize the signs that may indicate fatty acid deficiency. If obvious signs of fatty acid deficiency exist you should take immediate steps to correct this through modifying your child's fat intake. It may be necessary to consult a practitioner knowledgeable in nutrition. The signs of fatty acid imbalance include:

- Follicular hyperkeratosis (so-called "chicken skin" on the upper arms—this also may suggest beta-carotene insufficiency).
- Dandruff on scalp.
- Hair that is dry and unmanageable.
- Areas of leukoplakia.
- Nails that are brittle, fray easily, or won't grow.
- Areas of "alligator skin" (anywhere on the body).
- Patches of pale, lusterless skin on the cheeks.
- Dry ear wax or excessive production of ear wax.
- Allergies.
- Excessive thirst.
- Hyperactivity (ADD).

The Importance of Intestinal Bacteria

Before birth, the fetal intestinal tract is sterile, i.e., it contains no bacteria. The intestinal bacteria arrive in the newborn as a result of transit through the birth canal, during which time the child is exposed to the mother's fecal and vaginal bacteria. Following this, the child is exposed to microbes from the skin, the environment, and food. This is nature's way of ensuring that the infant digestive tract contains the organisms needed to function properly. The intestinal bacteria outnumber the human cells in the entire body.

The most common bacteria in the infant digestive tract are *Bifidobacterium bifidus*, *Lactobacillus acidophilus* and *Escherichia coli*. *Bifidobacteria* account for about 99 percent of the intestinal bacteria in breastfed infants. Bottle-fed infants have far lower fecal levels of *Bifidobacteria*. After the child has been weaned, the number of *Bifidobacteria* decline rapidly. Meanwhile, *E. coli* and *L. acidophilus* increase in number until *E. coli* predominates.

Each of these bacteria perform necessary functions in the child's intestinal tract. *B. bifidus* and *L. acidophilus* possess the following beneficial functions:

- Allow for an increased number of lymphocytes and larger lymph nodes.

- Increase the number of plasma cells and serum immunoglobulins.

- Contribute to increased phagocytic activity in macrophages. The macrophages of germ-free animals digest bacteria more slowly, suggesting that the gut microbes play a role in macrophage activity.[44]

- Produce organic acids and hydrogen peroxide which kill invading microbes, thereby protecting the body against infection from food-or water-borne pathogens.[45]

- Synthesize important B-vitamins such as niacin, pantothenic acid, pyridoxine, biotin, and folic acid.[46]

- Digest lactose and other dietary components, and play a role in the digestion and assimilation of milk.[47]

- Allow for better utilization of nutrients from food. Germ-free animals (lacking intestinal bacteria) experience far more pronounced symptoms if their diet is deficient in nutrients than if the gut flora is intact.[48]

- Encourage more efficient weight gain.[49]

- Participate in detoxification of some toxic compounds that enter the body via food or water, thus protecting us from a toxic environment.[50]

- Inhibit certain types of tumor growth.[51]

- Prevent the fungus *Candida albicans* from forming invasive germ-tubes.[52]

- Inhibit the growth of *C. albicans* in both the digestive tract and vagina. *Candida albicans* is the organism present in vaginal yeast infections and oral thrush.[53]

- Protect against many microbial pathogens such as *Salmonella*, *Shigella*, and virulent strains of *E. coli*.

- Produce organic acids that stimulate intestinal peristalsis, which in turn removes invading pathogens from the intestinal tract. (Peristalsis refers to the action of the intestinal muscles that moves the contents of the intestines forward.)

- Work in concert with the host immunological system (e.g., IgA).

In chapter 2, I said that antibiotics exert a pronounced adverse effect on the beneficial bacteria in the intestinal tract. You can see from the information above that the function of these bacteria is extremely important to the health of your child. Therefore, when antibiotics are being or have been used, it is important to reestablish these helpful bacteria in large numbers. This is accomplished by feeding the bacteria in some form to your child.

Supplementation of the diet with bacterial cultures has been used for centuries, most commonly as yogurt. Yogurt contains two main species of bacteria—*Streptococcus thermophilus* and *Lactobacillus bulgaricus*. *L. bulgaricus*, like *acidophilus*, is an acid-forming bacteria that digests lactose. It also inhibits harmful bacteria and parasites. This is one reason that consuming yogurt is associated with so many benefits. However, the bacteria found in yogurt, while helpful, are unable to establish a permanent colony. Because of this, the healing effects of yogurt are short-lived.

In contrast, *L. acidophilus* can become a permanent resident of the intestine by attaching tenaciously to the intestinal wall. In doing so, it prevents the attachment of many harmful organisms such as *Candida albicans* and *Giardia lamblia*. Today, some forms of yogurt contain viable cultures of *L. acidophilus*. However, the number of organisms is lower than in supplements.*

The best long-term benefit is to be derived from a combination of *L. acidophilus* and *B. bifidus*. Neither *L. acidophilus* nor *B. bifidus* are found naturally in foods. They are either obtained in supplement form or added to dairy products.

Who Might Need *Acidophilus* or *Bifidus* Supplements?

- Children with a history of oral thrush.
- Children with a history of diarrhea, constipation, or colic.
- Children known to have or suspected of having food allergies.
- Children with skin conditions such as eczema.
- Children believed to suffer from intestinal candidiasis.
- Infants born to a mother with a history of vaginal candidiasis.
- Hyperactive children where the hyperactivity appears to

---

*Yogurt is still an excellent food and can be used with great benefit provided your child is not sensitive to it. The point is that acidophilus or bifidus supplements yield better long-term results.

be associated with food allergy/sensitivity or digestive disturbance.

• Children with a history of antibiotic therapy.

• Children about to undergo antibiotic therapy.

• Children who have been bottlefed from birth or weaned before three months. All bottlefed children should receive bifidus daily.

• Children who have had solid foods introduced before three months of age.

• Children born by C-section.

• Children with recurrent tonsillitis.

• Children with recurrent otitis media.

• Children with a recent history of intestinal viral infection. (Enteric viruses generally reduce the fecal levels of acid-forming bacteria to near zero.)

• Children with known parasitic infections such as *Giardia lamblia* or *Entamoeba histolytica*.

How Do I Find a Quality *Acidophilus* or *Bifidus* Supplement?

Here are some guidelines that will be helpful in determining which *acidophilus* or *bifidus* supplement to buy.

1. These organisms are temperature-sensitive and must be refrigerated at all times. If you purchase it off the shelf (unrefrigerated), it is going to be less effective. Some companies will ship it in refrigerated containers upon request.

2. The number of viable organisms is important. Look for a product that specifically states the number of viable organisms. It should contain at least 1 billion or more. The label also should state the identifiable strain of organism since most of the research has been done on strains DDS1 and

NCFM. Other strains have not been as thoroughly tested for effectiveness.

3. Enteric coating of *acidophilus* or *bifidus* is an unnecessary process and serves only to reduce the number of viable organisms in the product. *Acidophilus* and *bifidus* are acid-loving organisms. Therefore, the environment of the stomach should not bother them appreciably unless the product contains a strain that is less hearty—something you're trying to avoid. Another problem with enteric coating is you can never predict if the coating will break down in time to insure maximum release of the organisms.

4. Sweet *acidophilus* milk contains living *acidophilus*, but in most cases, it is *Lactobacillus bulgaricus*—hearty, but it doesn't colonize the intestinal tract. In addition, the numbers are considerably lower than in a high-quality supplement, making the milk unsuitable in a treatment program.

   Sweet *acidophilus* milk would be acceptable as part of a maintenance program once reinoculation has been established (provided an allergy to casein does not exist).

5. Products are now available that include a variety of beneficial intestinal microbes in addition to the standard "acidophilus" and "bifidus." These include *Lactobacillus rhamanosus, L. bulgaricus, L. casei, L. sporogenes, Bifidobacterium longum* and *B. breve,* and others. A mixed culture such as this along with FOS can be a very helpful solution to imbalanced intestinal ecology.

6. Fructooligosaccharide (FOS) is a form of soluble fiber that is a preferred form of fuel for bifidobacteria. Using FOS can spur the growth of bifidobacteria and significantly improve the benefit derived from taking bifidobacteria. Some people with intestinal yeast overgrowth may react to FOS.

Dosage and Recommendations

1. ¼ teaspoon in ¼ glass of lukewarm water is frequently used to initiate therapy.

2. Dosage is often increased to ½ or 1 full teaspoon one to three times daily.

3. Take during mid-meal.

4. *Bifidus* is the recommended supplement for bottlefed infants.

5. When given concurrently with an antibiotic, *bifidus* is best given at times between the antibiotic. When sulfa drugs are used, the spacing should be two to three hours.[54]

6. Obtain a high-quality product—this is essential!

Note: If adverse reactions occur, they are usually due to one or more of the following:

1. Herxheimer reaction. This occurs when organisms are killed abruptly, resulting in a release of the toxic contents within their cell membranes.

2. Inferior product.

3. Casein or lactose intolerance.

Putting It Together

In this chapter I've described a number of home care treatments that work well. Obviously, you will not be using all of these on your child. So here are some basic guidelines that will help you decide how to proceed.

1. Approach your child's problem as though it is related to food or airborne allergies until proven otherwise (Food allergies will likely be more common.) This means following the guidelines in the section on allergies. Remove dairy products temporarily and watch for

improvement in your child's health. If allergies exist, remove the offenders from your child's diet or environment to the best of your ability. Adopt a strategy of rotation. Don't feed the same foods every day.

2. Assume there are nutritional needs that are not being met. This is especially true with essential fatty acids. Give essential fatty acids and other nutrients in the amounts listed.

3. Avoid known antagonists to good health including trans fatty acids, sugar, refined foods, and toxic metals. Reduce your child's intake of fruit juices, especially cold juices. When you give juice make sure it is fresh squeezed, not from concentrate. Follow the guidelines in chapter 7 that apply to your situation.

4. Choose a homeopathic medicine based on the symptoms of your child and the guidelines listed in the above section on homeopathy.

5. Use ear drops, nose drops, or acupressure to make your child more comfortable.

6. Give a *bifidus* supplement if your child falls into any of the categories listed in "Who Might Need *Acidophilus* or *Bifidus* Supplements?"

7. Take your child to the doctor if her condition does not respond within a reasonable amount of time. (See guidelines at the beginning of this chapter.)

8. Take comfort in the fact that many earaches resolve on their own. This is especially true if you take steps to improve immune function through good diet, nutrition, and lifestyle.

Chapter 7

Preventing Ear Infections in Your Child

Prevention encompasses two basic ideas. First, that disease can be prevented by considering the physical, chemical, and emotional needs of the individual child. And second, that illness already begun can be prevented from progressing by using effective home care or professional care practices. In this chapter, prevention strategies falling into the first category will be discussed.

Breastfeeding

Breastfeeding is perhaps the most effective means of preventing not only middle ear infection, but infections of all types. Dr. R.K. Chandra, in three separate studies, investigated the effect of breastfeeding on the incidence of infection and allergy. He demonstrated, in India, that breastfed infants had a lower incidence of otitis media and respiratory infections (and diarrhea, dehydration, and pneumonia) than did children who were not breastfed. In Canada, breastfeeding was again associated with a decrease in the occurrence of otitis media and respiratory infection.[1, 2]

Dr. Chandra also showed that when newborn siblings of children with allergic disease are exclusively breastfed for a minimum of six weeks, the number of allergic indicators, including lowered antibodies to cow's milk, are significantly reduced.[3]

The duration of breastfeeding also appears to have an impact on the development of otitis media. Finnish researcher Dr. Ulla

Saarinen followed 256 babies, born in the same three months, for one year. Of those breastfed for more than 6 months, only 6 percent had suffered an attack of otitis by the age of one year, in contrast to 19 percent of bottle-fed infants. Six percent of the children who had prolonged breastfeeding suffered four or more attacks of otitis media between one and three years of age, compared with 26 percent who had early introduction of cow's milk. Dr. Saarinen concluded that early and prolonged breastfeeding exerts a protective effect (against otitis media) that lasts up to three years.[4]

A recent finding lends further support to prolonged breastfeeding. Researchers found that breastfeeding protected against the development of otitis media, but that the risk increased four months after breastfeeding was discontinued. Approximately 12 months after breastfeeding was discontinued, the risk of developing otitis media was virtually the same as if the children had never been breastfed. This led researchers to conclude that "The risk of otitis media depends on the number of months a child is breastfed and the number of months that pass after breastfeeding is discontinued."[5] It seems to lend further support to cultural traditions in which mothers breastfeed for two to three years of age, ages at which children in Western cultures are particularly prone to otitis media.

Breastmilk even appears to prevent middle ear problems in children with cleft palate. Most children with cleft palate have difficulty suckling and are usually fed artificially (i.e. formula). They suffer inordinately from otitis media, require persistent antibiotic therapy, and often require surgery. Dr. Jack L. Paradise found that when mothers used a breast pump to gather their milk and then fed this to their children with cleft palate, the number of episodes of middle ear effusion was significantly reduced. Thirty-two percent of the breastmilk children were free of middle ear fluid at one or more office visits compared with roughly 3 percent of those fed cow's milk or soy formula.[6]

Breastmilk is high in an antibody called secretory IgA, something the child does not make in adequate amounts. Secretory IgA is a very important immune protein that protects against infection.

Breastmilk also contains proteins (called receptor analogues) that protect against attachment of bacteria. When these proteins are present, bacteria may exist in the environment, but their attachment is prevented. The ability of bacteria to attach is strongly associated with their ability to cause illness. Common ear-infecting bacteria such as *H. influenzae* and *S. pneumoniae* can be prevented from attaching by these proteins.[7]

An emerging story is the important role of breastmilk fatty acids in brain formation. Recent studies have shown that essential fatty acids arachidonic acid (AA) and docosahexaenoic acid (DHA) are crucial to brain development. Children who have been breastfed have been shown to have better visual acuity, random dot stereoacuity and matching ability than formula-fed babies. These improved visual abilities have been correlated with higher levels of DHA.[8] Another study showed higher IQ in breastfed children.[9]

I encourage mothers to breastfeed for a minimum of six months. Breastfeeding for one year is preferred. In many cultures, mothers breastfeed for three to four years. This is medically sound and culturally supported. In industrial cultures, support for this length of breastfeeding is not as broad. However, breastfeeding for several years is best for the child.

Concerns have been raised over the inability of human milk to supply adequate iron in children exclusively breastfed. However, the iron in breastmilk is sufficient to prevent anemia, for up to nine months. In addition, the mean hemoglobin concentration has been shown to be higher in breastfed infants than in iron-supplemented children at four and six months.

Please recognize that this section is not intended to bring guilt upon mothers who have chosen not to breastfeed or who have been unable to breastfeed. I realize that the decision to breastfeed is a very personal one that is complicated by mothers' working, lack of social support and other factors. Moreover, adoptive mothers do not have the opportunity to breastfeed. However, a rapidly growing mountain of evidence suggests that breastfeeding is critical to immune development and brain development and may have lasting implications into adulthood. Therefore, I cannot, in good conscience, fail to make a strong case for breastfeeding.

For parents who wish to augment their child's diet with increased levels of DHA I suggest a product called UltraCare for Kids. This is not an infant formula and should not be used as such. It is a hypoallergenic, rice-based nutrient formula with enhanced levels of omega-3 fatty acids including DHA.

Whatever length of time you choose to breastfeed, keep in mind that lactation is very nutritionally demanding for a mother. To insure that your baby continues to receive adequate amounts of zinc, iron, fatty acids and other nutrients, you must maintain a diet which is high in these nutrients. A multivitamin supplement (one that is free of sugar, wheat, dairy, yeast, additives, etc.) coupled with a balanced diet is an advisable way to replace the nutrients lost during lactation.

Avoid megavitamin supplementation or single nutrient supplementation during lactation. Not only do nutrients taken in excess go directly into the breastmilk, but some can even inhibit lactation. For example, mothers frequently need additional vitamin B6 during pregnancy and following delivery. However, if B6 is taken in excess (150–200 mg/day), it can inhibit lactation.

Because of the tendency for the breastmilk of American mothers to be deficient in fatty acids, I advise lactating mothers to take one perle of flax oil, one perle of a DHA oil, and one perle of evening primrose oil or borage seed oil daily, along with additional vitamin E. A general rule of thumb is .75 IU of vitamin E for every milligram of essential fatty acid.

Occasionally, breastfed infants will develop recurrent otitis media. When this occurs, it is usually due to a food (or foods) in the mother's diet to which either the mother or the child is allergic. The most common foods that trigger reactions in breastfed infants are dairy products, peanuts, and eggs. Challenge feeding tests can usually be used to identify sensitivities to foods. Once the offending food is identified, it can be eliminated from the diet. If challenge feeding (elimination-provocation) yields no clear results, your child may have a nutritional need that is not being met. This can sometimes be difficult to solve. In cases like this, make sure that fatty acid and zinc intake is sufficient. Finding a doctor knowledgeable in nutrition is important.

Feeding Position

Avoid feeding your baby a bottle while she is lying on her back in the crib, playpen, or anywhere else. Feeding in this position *increases* the likelihood that formula will reflux (or back up) into the eustachian tube. I advise mothers to treat their bottlefed baby as a nursing mother would treat her suckling infant. A nursing mother does not have the option of lying her child down (separately) while feeding. The mother and baby remain in close contact at all times. This provides not only a nourishing experience for the child, but a nurturing one for both mother and child. A mother who bottlefeeds her child should take the same opportunity to nurture by holding her child while feeding the bottle.

Preventing Airborne Allergy and Otitis Media

Reducing the level of airborne allergens in the home can be an important part of preventing recurrent earaches, especially (but not only) in children who have known airborne allergies. Here are some considerations:

Electrostatic Furnace Filter

These remove allergens and microbes from the air with electrically charged plates. The positively charged debris is attracted to the negatively charged plates, and the negatively charged debris is attracted to the positively charged plates. These can go a long way toward purifying the stale and polluted air in a home during winter. These filters have one major drawback—a fair amount of maintenance is required to keep the precipitators free of debris. But if they are well-maintained, electrostatic filters can reduce respiratory problems (including otitis) considerably.

These devices are also helpful in summer if central air conditioning is used. Electrostatic air cleaners are essential for children with known airborne allergies, but are recommended for any household since particulates in the winter or summer can irritate the mucous membranes of even healthy individuals.

Negative Ion Generator

These devices emit a stream of negatively charged ions that cause positively charged debris to precipitate out of the air (with the aid of a filter). Research I and my colleagues conducted with a Minnesota university showed negative ion generators coupled with filtration to be one of the most effective ways of removing bacteria, mold, fungi, and dust from the air. Negative ion generators are extremely efficient at removing cigarette smoke (although it is no substitute for the cessation of smoking).

Ion generators are practical in a room to room setting. They must be coupled with a filter to provide any real benefit.

Woodstoves and Fireplaces

These should be well-built with a source of outside air. A University of Michigan study showed that the incidence of upper respiratory problems was significantly greater in children living where woodstoves were used in the home. Fireplace centers can assist homeowners in the specifics of attaching an outside air source to their woodstove or fireplace. This is essential in all homes, not only in those where children exhibit illness.

In 1985, one of my patients lamented that each of his three children was sick with something nearly all winter long. Two of the boys had chronic recurrent ear infections and the third suffered from bronchitis. After questioning the father for some time, it appeared that the woodstove they were using might be responsible for his childrens' ongoing health problems. I suggested that he disconnect the woodstove (which was their primary source of heat) and use their backup system for the next month. Within two weeks, all children showed improvement. By the fifth week, things were back to normal for the family except for an occasional cold. This family had a woodstove that was inefficient and poorly ventilated. The gases and particulates that had built up inside the home as a result of burning were a source of constant upper respiratory irritation to the children.

It is advisable to have a negative ion generator operating in the room where your fireplace or woodstove is burning. This will help to filter most of the soot, smoke, and particulates that inevitably end up in the house because of burning.

Household Dampness

Damp areas should be eliminated and the sources identified. Mold and mildew are often imperceptible either by sight or smell, but can aggravate persistent middle ear problems in sensitive children. The bathroom, basement, and kitchen are the most likely areas.

Volatile Indoor Air Pollutants

In chapter 5, I described the manner in which volatile organic vapors can cause irritation of the upper respiratory tract and middle ear. The items that contribute to this should be identified and removed from the home. These include waxes, polishes, varnish, paint, cleaning solutions, old newsprint, and much more. The table listed in chapter 5 is a useful general guide to the substances containing volatile compounds.[10] For alternatives to some of the toxic products found in the home, I suggest you read *The Non-Toxic Home* and *Non-Toxic and Natural*, both by Debra Lynn Dadd.

Vacuum Cleaners and Carpeting

Dr. Edward Kenny, of the York Research Laboratory, claims that rugs and carpets test about 20 times dirtier than the average city sidewalk.[11] The carpet is where infants and toddlers spend most of their time, so ensuring a clean play area is crucial. Typical "bag filter" vacuum cleaners are notorious for moving more dust around the home than almost any other source. They are also a harbor for housemites, bacteria, and antigens. (See chapter 5.)

To solve this problem, many allergists recommend a "water vacuum" for cleaning homes. In a study by the Missouri State Medical Association, it was discovered that the Rainbow Vacuum (Rexair Corporation) can reduce the household dust concentration to one-fifth the amount that exists when ordinary bag-type vacuum cleaners are used. Another acceptable option is a central vacuum system with an outside exhaust.

Air-to-Air Heat Exchanger

These units function to bring fresh air into the home during the winter with only minimal heat loss. By continuously removing stale air and bringing in fresh, the number of air-borne irritants is reduced.

Air Travel

While not a significant contributor to otitis media, flying in an airplane can result in considerable distress for many children. Because of the rapid change in pressure, the eustachian tube sometimes does not open properly. To prevent problems with air travel, an infant should be nursed, given a pacifier, or given a bottle upon take-off and landing. Older children can be given a beverage to sip or gum to chew.

Smoking

The evidence linking smoking and childhood otitis media is indisputable. Cigarette smoke is among the most significant respiratory irritants found indoors. Its ability to cause otitis media in children is well documented. The solution for parents who smoke is to either quit smoking or smoke outside the home. If you choose to continue smoking in the presence of your child, first consider the adverse effects of smoking on the ears and then the added adverse effects of repeated antibiotics (to which your child will likely be subjected). Also consider that the alternative methods described in this book may be significantly *less* effective if you continue to smoke.

The Day Care Dilemma

The number of children spending time in day care grows each year. Health officials have estimated that approximately two-thirds of all preschool children and three-quarters of all school age children need some sort of child care while their parents work.[12] With this rise in day care usage comes and increased risk of illness to the children who participate.

Infants and toddlers in day care settings are twice as likely as those in home care to contract an illness that lasts more than 10 days, causes a fever of at least 102 degrees for three or more days, or requires medical attention.[13] For a variety of reasons, germs easily spread from child to child in the close quarters of the day care setting. A variety of infectious organisms have been isolated from day care workers and children. Among the most common are:[14]

- *Giardia lamblia*
- *Shigella*
- *Salmonella*
- *Escherichia coli*
- *Entamoeba histolytica*

- *Adenoviruses*
- *Rotavirus*
- *Haemophilus influenzae*
- *Streptococcus pneumoniae*

Dr. Stanley Schuman, of the Medical University of South Carolina, blames day care centers for "outbreaks of illness—diarrhea, dysentery, giardiasis, and epidemic jaundice—reminiscent of the pre-sanitation days of the 17th century."[15] A study published in 1984 revealed that children in day care centers were more than 12 times as likely to be infected with *Hemophilus influenzae* type b.[16] Another showed that day care children are 15 to 20 times more likely to contract giardiasis than children under maternal home care.[17]

Researchers at the University of Alabama found that 59 percent of day care children were shedding cytomegalovirus. Cytomegalovirus (CMV) was found on toys and other items frequently handled by children in the day care center. Based on antibody testing, it was estimated that between 70 and 100 percent of day care children were infected with CMV.[18]

A study reported in the *American Journal of Public Health* in 1988 compared children raised at home, raised in another home, and placed in nursery school or day care. The investigators in this study found that, compared to children reared at home, children in day care spent 30 percent more sick days in bed, while those raised in another home spent 19 percent more sick days in bed. Children in day care were also likely to spend more time in hospitals than children raised at home.[19,20]

A number of studies have shown that otitis media occurs more frequently in day care children than in children minded at home.[21,22] Drs. L. Birch and O. Elbrond compared the rate of otitis media in children minded exclusively at home with those spending time in day care. They found the occurrence of otitis media to be significantly higher in those attending day care centers. Moreover, long-lasting episodes of otitis media were found to be considerably more common among the children in day care centers.[23] A 1988 report in the *Journal of Pediatrics* revealed that hospitalization for myringotomy and tube placement occurred in 21 percent of the children in day care compared with only 3 percent of those in home care.[24]

Day care is here to stay. Many families require two incomes in order to survive. Certainly, many single parents would find it impossible to work or go to school without available day care for their children. Even the federal government has expressed its need to have mothers in the work force. However, the health implications of the growing day care situation are enormous. Public health officials are working to stem the rising tide of infections in day care children. At this stage there seems to be little progress. Some have recommended mass immunization of day care children, but this carries with it a host of social, philosophical, and medical implications.

Parents and day care providers should be aware of things they can do to reduce the spread of infectious disease. For parents, it is necessary to be aware of times when your child should be kept out of day care. For providers, it is important to know which children should be excluded or sent home. These are only first steps since the nature of the day care environment contributes to the spread of illness among children.

Recognize that otitis media is not considered a communicable disease in the strict sense. Yet, many of the conditions that predispose children to the development of middle ear effusion are considered communicable. The following guidelines are useful in determining when to exclude children from day care. For more information, contact your local community health department.

Guidelines For Excluding From Day Care

Children who have the following symptoms should be excluded from the child care setting until 1) a physician has certified the symptoms are not associated with an infectious agent or the child is no longer a threat to the health of other children at the center, or 2) the symptoms have subsided.

For the mildly ill child, exclusion should be based on whether there are adequate facilities and staff available to meet the needs of both the ill child and other children in the group.

FEVER
Axillary or *oral* temperature: 100 degrees F. or higher, or *Rectal* temperature: 101 degrees F. or higher; especially if accompanied by other symptoms such as vomiting, sore throat, diarrhea, headache and stiff neck, or undiagnosed rash.

RESPIRATORY SYMPTOMS
Difficult or rapid breathing or severe coughing:
—child makes high-pitched croupy or whooping sound after he coughs.
—child unable to lie comfortably due to continuous cough.

DIARRHEA
An increased number of abnormally loose stools in the previous 24 hours.
Observe the child for other symptoms such as fever, abdominal pain, or vomiting.

VOMITING	Two or more episodes of vomiting within the previous 24 hours.
EYE/NOSE DRAINAGE	Thick mucus or pus draining from the eye or nose.
SORE THROAT	Sore throat, especially when fever or swollen glands in the neck are present.
SKIN PROBLEMS	Rash—Skin rashes, undiagnosed or contagious. Infected sores—Sores with crusty, yellow or green drainage which cannot be covered by clothing or bandages.
ITCHING	Persistent itching (or scratching) of body or scalp.
APPEARANCE, BEHAVIOR	Child looks or acts differently: unusually tired, pale, lacking appetite. Confused, irritable, difficult to awaken.
UNUSUAL COLOR	Eyes or skin—yellow (jaundice) Stool—Gray or white Urine—Dark, tea-colored These symptoms can be found in hepatitis and should be evaluated by a physician.

Reprinted with permission from "Infectious Diseases in Childcare Settings: Information for Directors, Caregivers, and Parents or Guardians," prepared by the Epidemiology Departments of: Hennepin County Community Health, St. Paul Division of Public Health, Minnesota Department of Health, Washington County Public Health, Bloomington Division of Health. These guidelines are not to be considered all-inclusive. They are subject to ongoing revision as more information becomes available.

The Day Care Diet

Be aware of what your child is being fed while attending day care. Cheese, cold apple juice, and peanut butter sandwiches are common fare. However, consumption of these foods on a daily basis can irritate a toddler's digestive system and be a contributor to recurring illness. Determine the foods that best suit your child's specific needs and make arrangements to have this incorporated into your child's daily routine. Give your day care provider a list of foods that you wish your child to avoid. This may include foods to which your child is allergic or those that are not optimal for a child's digestion.

Dietary Considerations

Changing and improving dietary habits can be an important step in the prevention of recurrent earaches.

Early Introduction of Solid Foods

Solids should not be introduced before your child is six months of age. Earlier introduction solid food often contributes to health problems, including the development of allergies and earaches.

Recent evidence has linked the development of juvenile onset diabetes to ingestion of cow's milk in the first four months of life. A protein called bovine serum albumin (BSA) appears to cause the child's immune system to turn on the pancreas cells that produce insulin. Not every child is susceptible, but presently there is no way to tell who is at risk. Since BSA is passed through mother's milk it may be wise to avoid excessive milk consumption for the first several months of lactation.

Introduction of Solid Foods

When beginning to introduce solid foods into a baby's diet, it is important that only one food at a time be added. This way, if your child is sensitive to that food, you can identify it and avoid feeding it. Once your child's digestive tract has matured somewhat, you may wish to introduce the food again. Introduce the least aller-genic foods first. The first solids your baby eats should *not* be from among the most common offenders. These include:

- Dairy products.
- Wheat.
- Eggs.
- Chocolate.
- Citrus.
- Corn.
- Soy.
- Peanuts and other nuts.
- Shellfish.
- Sugar.
- Yeast.

Fruit Juice

Most children consume far too much fruit juice. A glass of juice is almost purely simple carbohydrate—in other words, sugar. Excess sugar leads to deficiencies in immune function, as described above. If you must give fruit juice, dilute it 1:1 with water, and don't give it cold out of the refrigerator. Most parents go to great lengths to make sure their baby's formula is warm, but think nothing of feed-ing a bottle of cold juice from the refrigerator. Cold juice can slow digestion in a child of any age.

Honey

Often, parents feel they are doing their child a service by feeding honey instead of sugar. This is a mistake if large quantities of honey are given, since honey contains the same sugar found in table sugar. There is an interesting phenomenon surrounding honey. When bee-keepers want to calm the hive, they mix a solution of sugar water and spray the bees. A solution of water and raw honey also has a calming effect on the bees. However, when pasteurized honey is used, all bees exposed will be found dead within 20 minutes.[25] It is unclear why this occurs, but it seems to suggest that raw honey may be a better dietary choice for humans than pasteurized honey. Almost all honey you find in the grocery stores is pasteurized. You have to look specifically for raw honey. A good place to start is a local food co-op or health food store.

Treat honey as you would any sugar and use it sparingly, especially if your child is ill. *Recognize that most doctors advise against feeding honey to children under one year.*

Sugar

A recent study showed that consumption of refined sugar was associated with low intakes of vitamin E. [26] Recall that vitamin E is important in immune function and for regulating inflammation. It is also low in the diets of children living in industrialized nations.

I treat this separately because sugar is added to nearly every type of packaged food available in stores. A study by Cheraskin and Ringsdorf has shown that when sugar is ingested, the ability of white blood cells to destroy bacteria can fall by as much as 60 percent.[22] Excessive sugar inhibits fatty acid metabolism (discussed in chapter 5) because it is high in calories but lacks the nutrients needed to make the enzymes work properly. High intake of sugar also increases the need for magnesium and increases the amount of magnesium excreted in the urine.[23, 24]

I suggest you read labels carefully. Any time sugar appears among the top five or six ingredients, don't buy the product.

Variety of Foods

Avoid feeding the same foods every day. Food sensitivity can be induced by overconsuming a given food every day for a long period. The solution is to rotate foods. Instead of feeding oatmeal every morning for breakfast, feed oatmeal one day, wheat cereal the next, fruit the next, and so on. With infants, rice is preferable to wheat.

If your child has known food allergies, don't feed those foods more than once or twice a week. When you do feed them, give only small amounts.

Cooked Food

Avoid feeding raw food to your infant. Fruits need not be cooked, but vegetables and other foods should be. Raw foods are more difficult to digest. They're also more apt to contribute to allergy. Also, cold food should not be fed to a child. When food is eaten cold the body must first warm it to almost 100 degrees (F) before it can be properly utilized. For an infant or child whose digestive system is immature, this can spell trouble.

Infant Formula

If you choose not to breastfeed, you should know a few things about infant formula. Powdered formula mix is higher in oxidized fats than is liquid formula. As I stated in chapter 5, oxidized fats in the diet can set the stage for inflammation and immune function problems. Some infant formulas contain aluminum in concentrations 30 to 100 times greater than that found in human milk. Aluminum is a toxic metalloid that has been implicated in brain and kidney damage.[30,31] For healthy infants this may not be a serious problem since the blood levels of aluminum following ingestion of formula are no higher than that of breastfed infants. At this time the issue is not clear.[32]

The greatest drawback of infant formula (following the absence of immune components) is the significant lack of the proper fatty acids. Most formula is too low in omega-3 and omega-6 fatty acids. Soy formulas are undesirable because of their low carnitine content.

Cow's milk causes allergic reactions in a large percentage of children. Cow's milk and most milk-based formulas (except Enfamil) contain insufficient amounts of the amino acid taurine. Taurine deficiency has been linked to the development of inflammatory conditions, which may be one reason cow's milk consumption gives rise to increased rated of infection and inflammation.

If you choose to feed cow's milk to your child under age two, use whole milk rather than skim or low-fat milk. Low-fat milk has a high protein-to-fat ratio, which is not suitable for infants and toddlers. Recognize that the American Academy of Pediatrics recommends that no child under age one receive whole cow's milk. Many physicians recommend no cow's milk at all. Also recognize that cow's milk products are found to be the most common provoking foods in children with middle ear problems and have been associated with an increased prevalence of type I diabetes in children at risk. Consumption of low-fat milk by children can cause kidney stress.

A category of formula that seems well-tolerated by many children is the protein hydrosylate. Protein hydrosylate refers to formula in which the cow's milk proteins have been predigested using and enzymatic process. Predigested milk proteins are less allergenic than intact cow's milk protein and therefore present less of a problem for potentially dairy-sensitive children. Examples of protein hydrosylate formulae include Nutramigen, Pregestimil, and Alimentum. Of these, Nutramigen was found to contain the lowest amount of intact bovine serum albumin, the protein that appears to trigger development of diabetes in some children. These types of formula are often more expensive, but are less allergenic options. Keep in mind that no formula on the market is even close to approximating the nutritional and immunologic value of breastmilk. In general, find a formula that contains DHA, LNA, and GLA or use a supplemental product that contains these fatty acids.

A product suitable for children over age one who are on solid food is called UltraCare for Kids. It is not an infant formula. It is designed as a supplemental high nutrient product that is hypoallergenic and contains no dairy or soy. An advantage of this product is that it contains the very important omega-3 fatty acid DHA. Recall that this is very important in brain development in infants and toddlers. UltraCare is available through health care professionals.

Essential Fatty Acids

As I mentioned in chapter 5, the amount of important omega-3 fatty acids in our diet has declined by 80 percent over the past 100 years. Omega-6 fatty acid consumption has remained relatively constant during this time, but because of other factors these fatty acids are sometimes not properly converted into prostaglandins. Therefore, a good prevention program consists of adding a small amount of omega-3 oils to your child's diet each day (especially if he has a history of allergies, skin problems, or infections).

The best vegetable source of omega-3 fatty acids is flax oil (not commercial linseed oil). I recommend the oil made by Spectrum Natural. (See resources.) It can be given ¼ teaspoon a day. I prefer flax seed oil that comes in perles since it is more stable and less subject to damage. Break open a perle and give the oil to your child rather than having them attempt to swallow it (unless over age six). Feeding walnut butter is a means to provide additional omega-3 fatty acids. By replacing peanut butter in the diet with walnut butter you also limit the intake of peanuts, a common food allergen.

An additional option is to give supplemental DHA (docosahexaenoic acid). DHA, as mentioned, is an omega-3 fatty acid important in nervous system function. It is available individually as a food supplement and as a component of some hypoallergenic rice-based drinks.

An ideal balance of supplemental essential fatty acids might include borage oil (for GLA), flax seed oil (for linolenic acid), and a special source of DHA. This would provide a reasonable balance of omega-6 and omega-3 fatty acids. If you wish to be more certain of the fatty acid status of your child a plasma or red cell (blood) fatty acid analysis can be ordered by your doctor. (See Appendix.)

Beginning in 1996, some formula manufacturers have added DHA to their infant formula. Additionally, some nutrition product companies offer DHA supplements that can be added to formulas, or given to a toddler or older child. (See Appendix for resources.)

As discussed in chapter 5, the enzyme necessary for proper conversion of fatty acids is inadequate in infants and is sometimes impaired in older children. So it may be helpful to give periodic doses of gamma-linolenic acid (GLA). Evening primrose oil is the best source of GLA. Borage oil is another good source. One perle can be given every other day in a prevention program. It is best to open the perle and give the oil rather than having your small child try to swallow it. Any formula-fed baby may need to be given GLA if he has health problems.

Never use the essential fatty acids I've discussed for cooking. They break down quickly when exposed to heat. They also break down when exposed to air. They should be stored in a brown bottle and refrigerated always. When taken out of the refrigerator, the amount needed should be taken and the cover quickly replaced.

Some suggest breaking open a capsule of vitamin E and placing the contents into your bottle of oil for better storage.

Always give additional vitamin E (5 to 25 I.U./day) when you feed your child essential fatty acids.

Trans Fatty Acids

Avoid feeding your child any of the non-essential fatty acids or foods containing partially hydrogenated oils. Foods to be avoided include:

- Cookies, pastries, doughnuts.
- Candy bars.
- Some crackers.
- French fries, potato cakes, chicken nuggets.
- Deep-fried fish sandwiches.
- Margarine.
- Vegetable shortening.
- Corn chips, potato chips.
- Malt balls (carob or chocolate).

Read labels! If the label says "may contain the following," be suspicious. If the "following" includes the words *partially hydrogenated*, avoid the product. Cottonseed oil, palm kernel oil, and coconut oil are also used frequently in packaged foods. Avoid these as well, since they are saturated fats that may interfere with the enzyme delta-6-desaturase, needed to convert fatty acids into prostaglandins. It might seem that eliminating these foods from the diet would take some fun out of life. Indeed, the list includes many childhood favorites. However, recurrent illness is no fun either. Any substantial reduction in the non-essential fats will go a long way toward improving your child's resistance to disease.

Drinking Water

Do not allow your child to drink soft water. Soft water contributes to magnesium loss and may contain excess sodium and aluminum. the most desirable alternatives are distilled water and water purified using a combination of carbon filtration and reverse osmosis.

Tap water often contains high levels of chlorine (for antibacterial purposes). The chlorine in tap water is believed by some to inhibit the beneficial bacteria in the intestines. In addition, when chlorine combines with organic matter present in water, it is converted to chloroform—a highly toxic substance.

Lead is another toxic element commonly found in tap water of older homes (before 1960). Lead leaches into the water from pipe joints that have been soldered using leaded materials (which is common). Since you cannot be sure if your water contains lead without having it tested, I recommend that you let the water run for three or four minutes every morning before using it. This will purge most of the lead from the water that has been standing overnight. Anytime your water has not been used for six or eight hours (or more), the water should be purged in this way.

Reduce Your Child's Intake of Canned Food

The average daily intake of tin (from canned food) is 200 mg/ day.[33] Tin is a known inhibitor of zinc and selenium, both of which play important roles in immune function and prevention of inflammation. Canned food is low in certain important nutrients such as folic acid and vitamin C, since these nutrients are dramatically affected by storage and processing. Canned foods used to contain measurable amounts of lead, but the practice of using lead solder in cans was stopped in the United States in 1992. Complete avoidance is not practical or necessary, but I would restrict the intake of canned foods.

Avoid Soft Drinks

I'm constantly amazed at the amount of soft drinks parents give to young children. The average soft drink contains 9 teaspoons of sugar. In addition, some (especially cola) contain high amounts of phosphoric acid, which binds with magnesium and pulls it out of the body. One 12-ounce can of cola contains 36 mg of phosphoric acid, which displaces 36 mg of magnesium. (Non-cola beverages often use ascorbic acid instead of phosphoric acid. Ascorbic acid does not have the same effect.) The importance of magnesium in fatty acid metabolism is described in chapter 5.

Intestinal Bacteria

Children who are formula-fed are often deficient in the bacteria *L. acidophilus* and *B. bifidus*. In breastfed babies, the numbers of these bacteria are high, but fall off once breastfeeding is stopped. Any child who has been on antibiotics probably needs *bifidobacteria*. Children in whom formula was introduced early in life also require *bifidus*. One teaspoon per day is an acceptable prevention dose.

Vitamins and Minerals

If your child consumes a diet consisting of whole foods, the need for additional vitamins and minerals should be minimal. A multivitamin supplement is usually all that is necessary unless there are obvious signs of nutritional deficiency. Be aware that many of the popular children's vitamins are loaded with sugar. I think this is unacceptable. When you choose a children's vitamin, read the label and be sure it contains no added sugar. Also be certain it contains no soy, yeast, wheat, milk, dyes, or other additives. This is especially important in a child with allergies.

What to Feed Your Child

Although this section contains "wisdom" about dietary practices that will help prevent ear infections, it is perhaps the Chinese to whom we should look for advice on proper eating. Acupuncturist Bob Flaws wrote in the *American Journal of Acupuncture* in 1989, "While interning at the Yue Yang Hospital with Dr. Chen [Li-chen] in 1984, I did not see a single case of pediatric otitis media." While gathered with senior physicians at the hospital, Flaws was asked what was the most common pediatric problem in the United States.

His response was "earache." The Chinese pediatric specialists agreed that earaches were not much of a problem in China.[34]

These doctors attribute the low rate of otitis media in Chinese children to the way food is cooked, combined, and introduced into their children's diets. In contrast, Chinese doctors studying in the West conclude that our children are being fed in a way that promotes the development of illness. I have to agree!

Chinese medicine has evolved through centuries of practice and observation. The dietary practices of the Chinese people have emerged from the same philosophical framework. As a student and practitioner of both Chinese and Western medicine I have learned that these time-honored traditions have an inherent wisdom and stability that in many ways surpasses our own. In my opinion, following the general principles of Chinese dietary practices can have a substantial impact on the health of children in the West.

It is beyond the scope of this book to discuss the details of food preparation and combining. For more information on Chinese dietary practices I suggest you read *Prince Wen Hui's Cook: Chinese Dietary Therapy* by Bob Flaws. For a Western perspective on diet and nutrition that includes food lists, menus, and other valuable dietary recommendations, I suggest you read *Superimmunity for Kids* by Leo Galland, M.D., and *Healing with Whole Foods* by Paul Pitchford.

Minor Injuries

In chapter 5, I described how biomechanical problems may lead to the development of middle ear problems in your child. Biomechanical problems can be identified and corrected at any time following an injury, but are best corrected soon after the injury occurs and before ear problems arise.

Following Birth

Following the birth of your child is the optimum time to have him examined for biomechanical problems of the spine.

An examination for biomechanical problems of the spine is essential:

- If the birth has been particularly long and difficult.

- If forceps or vacuum extraction have been used to assist delivery.

- If there are sensory or motor problems of the head and neck.

- In cases of infantile torticollis (where the child's head appears to be fixed in or favoring one direction).

- Where chronic infections of the upper respiratory tract exist from birth (including chronic stuffiness or sinus congestion).

Examination of the spine is advised:

- After every birth. Even the normal forces of uterine contraction can disrupt the delicate spinal biomechanics of a newborn.

Following Injury

Any slip or fall has the potential to cause disruption in the normal function of the spinal biomechanics. Those which are more serious are obviously also the ones that have a greater likelihood of contributing to problems. Even minor falls can disrupt the spinal mechanics enough to affect the middle ear and surrounding tissues.

Examination is essential:

- When your child has taken a serious fall such as down the stairs, on the ice, off the changing table, or off the couch.

- If your child complains of headache or neck stiffness following a fall (especially if the complaints last for more than a few days).

- If your child complains of ringing in the ears or dizziness following a fall.

Examination is recommended:

- Whenever you sense that something is not quite right following a fall. If you notice behavior changes, change in posture, change in eating habits, change in hearing, etc., you should consider having your child examined.

An examination for biomechanical problems of the spine is typically done by a doctor of chiropractic or doctor of osteopathy. (Both are licensed to practice in all 50 states.) Don't be surprised if you take your child into your family medical doctor and he declares your child to be free of any problems following a fall. He is trained to look for pathology. He will check reflexes, check for fractures, check for concussion, and for any other signs that would suggest serious damage. Your medical doctor is not looking for functional changes in the mechanics of the spinal column. The chiropractor or osteopath, while also checking for signs of more serious injury, will examine for changes in spinal biomechanics.

Treating Colds and Nasal Congestion

Roughly one-half of all middle ear problems are preceded by colds, nasal congestion, or another upper respiratory problem. Thus, an important preventive measure is to treat these conditions quickly before they begin to involve the middle ear. Because most of these conditions are viral in origin, allopathic medicine lacks an effective therapy. This is where homeopathic medicine is often at its best.

When your child develops a cold, it will be helpful to consider the other preventive measures described in this chapter. In the homeopathic care of cold, there are several remedies you will need to consider.

Homeopathic Single Remedies

Aconite

Used in the first 24 hours of a cold that is due to exposure to cold or wind. Often associated with high fever. Thirst and restlessness are usually present. A hoarse, dry, croupy cough that comes on suddenly may be present. A child will often experience fear, anxiety, and worry. They do not want to be touched. The mucous membranes are dry and the nose is stopped up. If there is nasal discharge, it is slight and watery. Occasionally, nasal discharge is bloody. Earache may be present.

Symptoms are worse: from dry, cold winds, tobacco smoke, in a warm room, and in evening and night.

Symptoms are better: in open air.

Allium cepa

Indicated when there is much sneezing associated with watery eyes and a runny nose. The nasal discharge tends to be clear, watery, and offensive. It is irritating to the upper lip and increases when entering a warm room. The eyes frequently burn from the profuse tearing. However, the tears do not irritate the skin around the eyes. Earache and shooting pains in the eustachian tube may occur. *Allium cepa* is commonly associated with hoarseness and a tickling sensation in the throat. This remedy is often used to treat the symptoms of hay fever.

Symptoms are worse: in warm room, toward evening.

Symptoms are better: in a cold room and open air.

Antimonium tartaricum

A useful remedy for coughs that come on gradually and are associated with rattling of mucus with little expectoration. These children are drowsy and weak. The face is cold, blue, and pale. There is often quivering of the chin and trembling throughout the body. *Antimonium tart* is used in the latter stages of respiratory problems that do not improve. These children often require medical attention.

Symptoms are worse: from warmth, lying down at night, damp cold weather, and in evening.

Symptoms are better: from expectoration and sitting up.

Arsenicum album

There is a profuse, watery nasal discharge with sore, burning nostrils. The nose feels stopped up. The eyes, which may be swollen, burn from offensive tears. This is a useful remedy for different types of coughs. There is burning in the chest. The cough may be worse after midnight or while lying on the back. Respiration is often accompanied by wheezing. Exhaustion, restlessness, and symptoms that are aggravated at night are important signs that *Arsenicum* is needed. These children are anxious and fearful. High fever is common.

Symptoms are worse: in a cold room, from cold or wet weather, and after cold food or drink.

Symptoms are better: from heat, warm drinks, and elevating the head.

Belladonna

This remedy is used in the early stages of a cold. The illness usually comes on rapidly with little warning. It is usually associated with hot, red skin, flushed face, glaring eyes, restless sleep, and hypersensitivity of all senses. The throat is hot and dry with swollen tonsils. Earache is common with *Belladonna*. There is hoarseness and dryness of the mucous membranes of the nose, throat, and trachea. There is usually fever present, but the skin is dry. There is commonly no thirst. The emotional symptoms are important with *Belladonna*. The child is almost unaware of what is going on around her. The acuteness of her senses may cause her to be agitated and furious, which may lead to outbursts of hitting or biting. These children may have fears of imaginary things, hallucinations, and delirium. The pupils are dilated.

Symptoms are worse: from touch, noise, draft, light, odors, and lying down.

Symptoms are better: by sitting semi-erect.

Euphrasia

Symptoms are almost the reverse of *Allium cepa*. The nasal discharge is non-irritating. The eyes, which seem to water constantly, produce tears that are highly irritating. There may be a mild cough.

Symptoms are worse: in evening, indoors, in a warm room (although the nasal symptoms are made worse in open air, in the morning and from lying down).

Ferrum phosphoricum

Ferrum phosphoricum is used both for colds and otitis media. This remedy is indicated in the early stages of a cold. It is commonly used in anemic children (although this is not a prerequisite) or after *Belladonna* has failed to give relief. There is tickling in the chest accompanied by a hard, croupy cough.

Symptoms are worse: at night and from touch.

Symptoms are better: with cold applications.

Gelsemium

There is an irritating watery nasal discharge. The hallmark of this remedy is chills running up and down the spine. Pervading the child is a general sense of sluggishness, heaviness, and muscular weakness. The cold comes on gradually. Breathing is slow and labored.

Symptoms are worse: in damp weather.

Symptoms are better: in open air and with motion.

Hepar sulphuricum

This is also an important remedy for otitis media. It is used in the latter stages of a cold when the nasal discharge has become thick, yellowish, and offensive. These children are easily irritated and are hypersensitive to touch. The voice may be lost when exposed to dry, cold air. The cough is loose, rattling, and commonly worse in the morning. This child is so sensitive to cold that a hand or foot exposed from beneath the covers causes aggravation of the cough.

Symptoms are worse: from dry cold winds, cold foods, or the slightest draft.

Symptoms are better: from warmth, humidity, and after eating.

Kali bichromicum

Kali bic is not a typical cold remedy but is an extremely valuable remedy for sinus congestion. Pain is around the root of the nose. Nasal discharge is thick, ropy, and greenish-yellow. Violent sneezing is common.

Symptoms are worse: with cold (air and drink).

Symptoms are better: with warmth and pressure.

Natrum muriaticum

The child awakens with much sneezing. Heavy nasal discharge, described as having a raw egg-white appearance, is present. Small eruptions or vesicles form around the lips. The lips and corners of the mouth are dry, ulcerated, and cracked. A crack in the middle of the lower lip is sometimes seen. These children are irritable, weepy, and wish to be alone. Their symptoms may be aggravated when one attempts to console them.

Symptoms are worse: from noise, consolation, lying down, heat, talking, and in a warm room.

Symptoms are better: from cold bathing, lying on right side, going without regular meals, and in open air.

Nux vomica

This remedy is used after exposure to dry, cold weather. However, the symptoms do not come on as rapidly as with *Aconite*. Heavy nasal discharge is fluid during the daytime, but stuffed up at night. Discharge may alternate from left to right nostril. There is hoarseness with a sensation of scraping in the throat. *Nux* children are irritable, sensitive and do not like to be touched. They are sensitive to noises, odors, and light. When a cough is present, it is worse after eating or upon waking. The cough is often dry and hacking. These children are greatly sensitive to cold.

Symptoms are worse: from touch, dry weather, cold, after eating, after mental work, and in the morning.

Symptoms are better: in the evening, while at rest, and after warm drinks.

Pulsatilla

This medicine is useful in acute otitis media but is also valuable for colds. There is thick, bland, yellowish-green discharge, sometimes accompanied by a dry or loose cough. There tends to be a dry cough in the evening and at night. In the morning there is a loose cough with copious expectoration of mucus. The nose is often stuffed at night. The child is weepy, easily discouraged, and melancholy. He is frequently feverish, but also thirstless. Symptoms improve markedly when he is outdoors. This child likes the head held high and often desires to sleep with more than one pillow.

Symptoms are worse: from heat, lying down, exertion, after eating, toward evening, and in a warm room.

Symptoms are better: with motion, cold applications, cold food and drink, and in open air.

Rhus toxicodendron

The nasal discharge is thick and yellow-green. The nose feels congested. A tickling sensation behind the breastbone is often accompanied by a dry, teasing cough from midnight until morning. *Rhus tox* is indicated for children who feel better when moving about. The remedy is often needed when there is itchiness of the skin.

Symptoms are worse: from cold, wet, rainy weather; during sleep, when lying on back, and at night.

Symptoms are better: from warm, dry weather; motion, walking, change of position, and warm applications.

Spongia

This is an important remedy for coughs that are dry, barking, and croupy. The cough usually improves after eating or drinking, especially warm drinks. There may be profuse nasal discharge alternating with blockage. These children are anxious and fearful. Any form of excitement aggravates their cough. They may awaken in the middle of the night with a fearful suffocating sensation.

Symptoms are worse: from wind, lying down, excitement, and before midnight.

Whenever a cough or cold becomes severe or is associated with vomiting, shortness of breath, or difficulty breathing, your physician should be consulted.

*   *   *

It is not possible to prevent the development of illness entirely. This is especially true in children because they are new creatures of this world. Every encounter with a strange bacterium or virus must by design arouse the defenses. This frequently manifests in symptoms that appear for a short time and then disappear, the battle having been won. This process is an essential part of developing the immune recognition system. This type of illness is expected. The illness we hope to prevent is that which is recurrent or that which lingers, gradually taking the strength from the sick child.

Chapter 8

Alternative Treatment:
Some Solutions

There is no longer any doubt about the value of incorporating traditional medicine into modern health care.[1]
Olayiwola Akerele, World Health Organization

Childhood otitis media is often as frustrating for doctors to treat as it is for parents to endure. There are those within medicine who are confident that the current state of treatment is effective and safe. Moreover, the public generally believes that there is a consensus among doctors regarding the safety, efficacy, and application of these methods. A look at the evidence presented in chapters 2 and 3 suggests, however, that there are many voices of dissension regarding the treatment of otitis media. Recall the following remarks by respected investigators in the fields of pediatrics and otolaryngology:

"The treatment of recurrent otitis media remains an unresolved problem."[2]

"There is no consensus of opinion regarding effective medical treatment of secretory otitis media."[3]

". . . secretory otitis media is a self-limiting disease, which is not affected by any of the current methods of treatment."[4]

"Otitis media with effusion . . . appears to be more common *since* the widespread use of antibiotics."[5]

What do these statements imply about the current state of treatment of otitis media? At the very least, they suggest that there is room for improvement—a niche which holistic methods might arguably fill. At best, comments such as these should cause us to consider fundamental changes in the clinical management of otitis media. It may be time to step back and reassess the problem. It may be time to embrace the holistic viewpoint. It may indeed be time to take a serious look at the holistic models already in place and determine what role they may play in the effective management of a problem in urgent need of solutions.

In this chapter are presented the most common and most effective methods used in the holistic management of otitis media. Based on anecdotal evidence and clinical case studies, the methods described below have been shown to have significant value in the care of otitis media. Admittedly, there is not sufficient scientific research on these methods at present. It is my hope that this chapter will serve as the foundation upon which further investigation into alternatives is based.

Using This Chapter

This section is intended primarily for health practitioners who want access to a resource for the care of otitis media. While this section is written for clinicians, there is a wealth of information useful to parents. Without a clinical background, however, it may be difficult to make practical use of the information.

In providing this information, I assume that:

- Anyone using this information has formal training in the health sciences.

- Anyone attempting to manage otitis media conduct an otoscopic examination (and a complete physical exam) on each child before engaging in any form of treatment. And that such persons be aware of the diagnostic implications of the various findings on otoscopic examination.

- Anyone using this information has training in one or more of the specialties described below.

- ·Anyone managing otitis media be fully aware of the potential for complications and the signs and symptoms associated with those complications.

Alternative Treatment Methods Described

The methods of management described below have been established based on clinical observation. They have been compiled from a variety of sources. To my knowledge, they have not been subjected to double-blind, placebo-controlled study in otitis media. Descriptions of each form of therapy are provided to show the detailed approaches used to treat otitis media and to serve as a background for those wishing to know more about specific diagnosis and treatment.

Information in this chapter is presented for educational purposes only. It is not to be construed as recommendation for treatment and is not intended to replace the clinical judgment of the physician. No claims of the ability to cure otitis media are made. Moreover, the information contained in this chapter should not be viewed as all-inclusive. Although I have attempted to provide a wide survey of the alternative methods used to manage otitis media, there may be others I have omitted.

The benefit of the methods described below is that they can be used to successfully treat constitutional weaknesses that typically predispose children to the development of otitis media. A profound example of recovery using holistic methods was reported to me by Dr. Martha Benedict. She describes the case of a two-year-old boy with recurrent otitis media. The boy had been on repeated antibiotics for some time. His infections had persisted for so long that the eardrum had almost completely dissolved. A look into the ear canal revealed virtually no eardrum. The ear ossicles were directly visible. The child's otolaryngologist began talk of surgically implanting a prosthetic eardrum.

Dr. Benedict began her treatment, which consisted of botanical medicine and dietary management. She described the child's diet as full of sugar and white flour. After several months of treatment, the earaches began to subside. What's most remarkable about this case is that Dr. Benedict observed a gradual regeneration of the eardrum. Over time, the eardrum was almost completely restored by natural means. I share this story not to imply that eardrums can be regenerated by diet and herbs, but to illustrate the remarkable healing ability of the body once constitutional weaknesses are overcome.

Listed below are six forms of alternative treatment currently used to manage otitis media. The philosophical and scientific basis behind each method of treatment is thoroughly described elsewhere and will not be presented here.

The six methods are:

- Allergy Management.
- Homeopathic Medicine.
- Manipulation.
- Acupuncture.
- Botanical Medicine.
- Clinical Nutrition.

Allergy Management

The clinical management of allergy is complex. To address it in sufficient depth would require another book the size of this one. It would, therefore, be presumptuous of me to attempt a detailed discussion of clinical allergy management. I have chosen instead to comment on the importance of addressing constitutional weaknesses in the child and outline the forms of allergy tests currently available.

The Constitutional Approach

Constitution refers to the child's (or any person's) general level of health. It takes into consideration his lifestyle, environmental influences, history of past illness, heredity, and even parental history of illness. Constitutional treatment is directed toward the management of these areas and toward restoring vigor to the body systems that are weak, damaged, or poorly functioning. Constitutional treatment is, therefore, not considered acute care. The use of constitutional treatment can take place alongside acute care.

Constitutional care also might be viewed as any effort to correct underlying metabolic problems. In this section, I will briefly address some underlying metabolic considerations in approaching the management of both airborne allergy (or hypersensitivity) and food allergy (or hypersensitivity). This is not intended to be a practical discussion, but more of a survey.

Indoor Air Pollution and Hypersensitivity

Vapors from chemicals such as benzene, toluene, and formaldehyde are found with increasing regularity in the air inside our homes. These compounds can cause mucous membrane inflammation in the eyes, ears, nose, throat, and lungs of most individuals exposed. In individuals sensitive to these compounds, severe hypersensitivity or allergic reactions can occur with exposure to only tiny amounts of such vapors. This includes adverse reactions of the immune system.

To deal with these compounds, the body has several separate defensive systems in place. One is the mixed function oxidase system (MFO), and another is the antioxidant defense system. When exposed to airborne pollutants, these systems go to work converting the chemicals into usually harmless substances that can be eliminated from the body. Some chemicals are converted into substances more toxic than those originally inhaled. Many compounds act as free radicals (discussed in chapter 5). The demands placed on the defensive system are considerable, but not overwhelming.

When exposure to such substances occurs over time—which happens in cases of urban air pollution or indoor air pollution—the defensive systems are overwhelmed and the antioxidants are depleted. What the body must do is shift, or shunt, its defensive platoons to those areas of the body that are receiving the greatest exposure. In our example, this is the lungs since the substances are breathed. By shifting defenses to the lungs, the body, in essence, reduces its defenses in other areas.[6]

The problem is that we are being exposed to similar substances through the food and water. This is especially true when diets are high in oxidized fats, or trans fatty acids. When diets are deficient in the raw materials—nutrients—needed to make the defensive systems work, the damaging effects of exposure to toxic substances are amplified.

What this means is that there may be an ever-increasing number of children sensitive to a wide variety of substances in their environment. Continued low-level exposure to toxic substances coupled with inadequate dietary intake of the vitamins and minerals needed to metabolize these substances may lead to increased reactivity to the environment (food, pollens, chemicals, etc.), greater immune compromise, susceptibility to infection, and susceptibility to inflammation.

Food Allergy and Intolerance

Many doctors argue that the incidence of food allergy is rising rapidly. Some contend that the rise is due to the increasing use of refined foods that are low in nutrients. Others contend that the overuse of antibiotics triggers serious imbalance in the intestinal ecology, resulting in inflammation and susceptibility to parasitic invasion. Yet others believe that toxic substances in the environment disrupt the metabolic machinery required to metabolize dietary macro and micronutrients. It is my opinion that the interplay of these and other factors probably contribute to the increasing incidence of food allergy in contemporary society.

How might this occur? Ours is an overconsumptive society. We know that overconsumption can lead to the development of food intolerance. This can occur when foods are consumed in large amounts or with high frequency. When overconsumption of refined foods occurs, a situation of high caloric intake coupled with low nutrient density exists. The result is insufficient nutrients to metabolize the ingested calories. The body must then rely on its reserves of these nutrients to drive the enzymes needed to metabolize such foods. Obviously, this cannot continue for long or the body's nutrient reserves will be depleted—especially in the case of water-soluble nutrients.

Added to this is the overconsumption of antibiotics. Whether our antibiotics are consumed for therapeutic reasons or through the food supply, the effects on digestion and metabolism can be significant. Inflammation, parasitic infestation, and food allergy have been linked to antibiotic overuse. Antibiotic use is linked to the so-called "leaky gut syndrome." In this syndrome, the intestinal lining has become thin and porous due to inflammation. The increased porosity of the gut leads to an increased uptake of incompletely digested proteins (or IBPs, discussed in chapter 5). The IBPs are absorbed intact and reacted upon by circulating lymphocytes in the blood. Thus, an allergic response to foods can occur from antibiotic overuse. until the intestinal integrity is restored, reactivity to foods continues.

How does one restore intestinal integrity? This is a complex issue that is not fully understood. We do know that nutrients such as vitamin A, beta-carotene, zinc, folic acid, vitamin E, and essential fatty acids are all vital to the rebuilding of the intestinal mucosa. Unfortunately, when intestinal inflammation exists, there is often reduced absorption of nutrients. Feeding a diet already low in nutrients will not encourage intestinal healing or reduction of food allergies. Therefore, some form of nutritional supplementation and dietary change is needed.

Then there is the problem of intestinal bacteria. When the colon is overrun with coliform bacteria or parasites such as *Candida albicans* or *Giardia lamblia,* these organisms must be dealt with before any restoration of intestinal integrity can occur. This usually involves anti-parasitic agents, nutrients, and reinoculation of the bowel with *Lactobacilli.* Food allergy occurs with great frequency when intestinal lactobacillus levels are low.

Heavy metals, such as lead and mercury, are yet another factor that may interfere with proper metabolism and contribute to the development of food allergy. Lead binds strongly with enzymes throughout the body. When lead binds with digestive enzymes, the enzymes become inactivated. In this state, the enzymes cannot carry out their task of breaking down food properly. The result is impaired digestion, impaired absorption, and development of food allergy.

Lead has also been shown to have an adverse effect upon immune function.

When dietary fiber intake is low, the transit of food through the digestive tract is slowed. When this occurs, partially digested food resides in the intestine for much longer than normal. This creates an environment in which intestinal bacteria can begin to putrefy the contents of the intestine. As this occurs, the pH of the gut changes, which results in an environment that often favors the growth of pathogenic bacteria at the expense of *Lactobacilli* and other beneficial organisms. One consequence is the development of food intolerance.

The above discussion only touches on the complexity of what must be considered in the management of allergy. The management of airborne allergy often requires changes in the child's immediate environment to reduce exposure to the offending agents. This is a beginning. Nutritional status also must be carefully evaluated. I've observed a direct link between the severity of airborne allergy and the presence of food allergy. When food allergy is properly managed, problems with airborne allergy frequently improve.

The management of food allergy (or hypersensitivity) begins with the identification of offenders. No matter which approach is taken, it is always helpful to reduce the intake of offending foods for a time. At the very least, foods should be rotated. This is especially true in pan-sensitive individuals who react adversely to nearly everything they eat. Often, simply removing cow's milk from the diet is enough to significantly reduce the occurrence of otitis media.

In food-allergic individuals, the intestinal function must be evaluated. This involves understanding bowel transit times, possible parasitic infection, nutritional status, enzyme activity, stool composition, absorption, and much more. The diet must be carefully evaluated to detect any significant imbalances in macronutrient or micronutrient intake.

Methods of Allergy Testing[7]

The methods described below are currently used to identify allergy to various substances.

Skin Testing (scratch test): Used to identify IgE-mediated reactions. The skin is pricked with a "scarifier" through a drop of antigen-containing solution. The skin is then observed for the development of characteristic reactions that include varying degrees of swelling and redness.

Radioallergosorbent Test (RAST): IgE-RAST detects antigen-specific IgE, type I immediate hypersensitivity. IgG ELISA detects delayed sensitivity reactions.

Intradermal Cutaneous Test: Used to identify immediate hypersensitivity reactions. The antigen is injected into the superficial layers of skin. The skin is observed for characteristic reactions.

Elimination-Provocation: Used to identify food allergy and hypersensitivity, i.e., food intolerance. (Allergy and hypersensitivity cannot be differentiated using this test.) Performed by putting the patient on an oligo-antigenic diet for one week, then challenging, one at a time, with suspected food antigens. A simplified version of this test can be done at home.

Lactulose-Mannitol Test for Permeability. As discussed in chapter 5, lactulose-mannitol challenge can determine whether excessive permeability to small molecules exists. There is increasing evidence that this test is a useful marker for food intolerance.

Of the above tests, elimination-provocation (EP) is the most reliable since it identifies both allergy and hypersensitivity (although it does not differentiate). Its chief drawbacks are that it: 1) takes days to weeks to complete, 2) requires patient motivation and compliance, potentially limiting the number of foods that can be tested, 3) does not give a clear indication of the degree of reactivity, and 4) is difficult to test for reactivity to additives and chemicals found in food (although, thus far, no tests are particularly successful at this). In spite of these drawbacks, EP is one of the most acceptable, reliable, and cost-effective assessment tools available for identifying food intolerance. It is advisable to use some form of EP in conjunction with laboratory tests.

Homeopathic Medicine

There are two basic considerations in the homeopathic management of otitis media. First, acute otitis media is managed using remedies that are selected based on their similarity to the acute syndrome. (See chapter 6.) While some of these remedies may be useful in chronic otitis media, they are specifically useful in acute otitis media. Second, chronic otitis media is believed to arise out of a fundamental weakness in the child's constitution or out of suppressive therapeutic intervention. In these cases, the homeopathic remedy is selected after an extensive evaluation of the complete symptom picture of the child. During the course of constitutional care, an acute flare-up of otitis media may occur. The doctor may then choose to treat the acute episode with an "acute" remedy and resume constitutional care once the episode has subsided.

Stephen Messer, N.D., has extensive experience in the homeopathic management of otitis media. At a 1986 conference on homeopathic medicine, he presented a lecture entitled "Homeopathy and Otitis in Children." In his address, Dr. Messer described in detail the process of decision-making that goes into selecting the appropriate remedy.* The following diagnostic categories form a basis for Messer's approach.[8]

Otitis Media Without Effusion: Redness of the tympanic membrane with normal mobility. There is no fluid.

Acute Otitis Media: Same signs as above. In addition, there is suppuration in the middle ear, and decreased mobility of the tympanic membrane.

---

*An audio tape of this lecture is available through Homeopathic Educational Services. See resources.

Otitis Media With Effusion: Serous fluid or pus lies behind the tympanic membrane. Mobility of the tympanic membrane is limited. There is often an absence of other symptoms.

Chronic Otitis Media: Chronic discharge of fluid, often pus, from the middle ear.

In otitis media without effusion and acute otitis media, the process of remedy selection is rather straightforward (although it still requires an evaluation of the child's general symptom pattern). First, a diagnosis of the child's condition is made based on otoscopic findings. Once the diagnosis is made, you refer to the appropriate flow chart (figures 15, 16, and 17).[9] For example, if you diagnose otitis media without effusion, the first question you ask is, is there a fever of more than 103 degrees? If the answer is "yes," you go to the next level of questioning. In this case, is the face bright red? If the answer is "no," the remedy is *Pulsatilla*. If the answer is "yes," you determine if the child is agitated and restless. Using this progression of logic, the correct remedy can be selected. The same type of process is used in acute otitis media. These flow diagrams are especially useful in small children, since small children can rarely communicate specifics about their pain.

In otitis media with effusion and chronic otitis media, Messer has observed that there is a hierarchy of remedies that must be considered. Remedies listed at the top of the hierarchy are those more commonly used in chronic otitis media. Those at the bottom are less frequently used, but no less important. Since chronic otitis media requires constitutional care, the hierarchy should be considered as a guide. The doctor must then research the *materia medica* for the remedies that fit the individual child.

Otitis media with effusion and chronic otitis media often occur as a result of repeated doses of antibiotics or because of an underlying constitutional weakness. In either case, remedies are required that are deep acting and can stir a response in a suppressed immune system. Occasionally, a child treated for chronic otitis media may get worse for a period before improving. This is because: 1) chronic

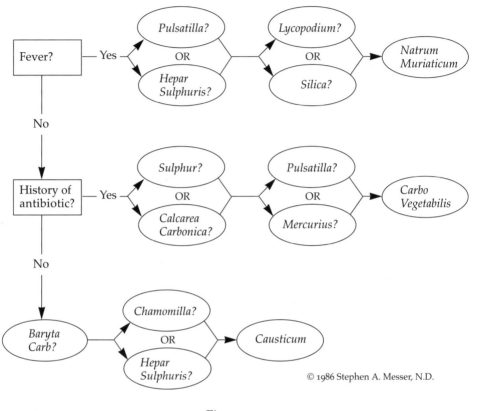

Figure 15
Acute Otitis Media

otitis media often occurs with only minimal symptomatology, thus any change tends to appear as an aggravation, and 2) a deep-acting remedy frequently arouses the body defenses sufficiently to begin acting against an ongoing infection. This type of response is not cause for alarm, but should be monitored closely. Communication with the parents of such a child is important.

The remedies described below are those most frequently used in chronic otitis media or otitis media with effusion. Recognize that remedy selection is not-clear cut in these children. When ear discharge occurs, the type of discharge is an important indicator in

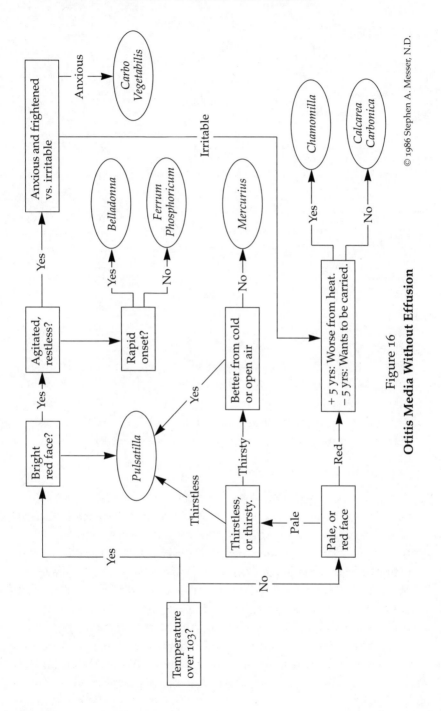

Figure 16
Otitis Media Without Effusion

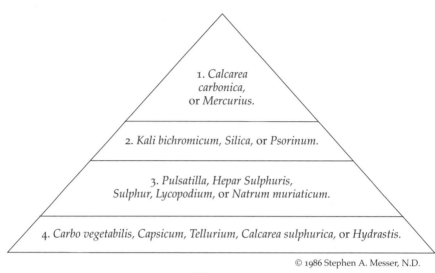

1. *Calcarea carbonica,* or *Mercurius.*

2. *Kali bichromicum, Silica,* or *Psorinum.*

3. *Pulsatilla, Hepar Sulphuris, Sulphur, Lycopodium,* or *Natrum muriaticum.*

4. *Carbo vegetabilis, Capsicum, Tellurium, Calcarea sulphurica,* or *Hydrastis.*

© 1986 Stephen A. Messer, N.D.

Figure 17
Chronic or Recurrent Otitis Media

remedy selection. However, children with chronic otitis are frequently asymptomatic, so ear signs and symptoms may be of limited value. In addition, silent forms of otitis media such as these may harbor complications. It is necessary to be alert for signs of meningitis, mastoiditis, and other potential problems. Anytime complications are threatening or present, a specialist should be consulted.

Dosage and Potencies

A method of prescribing known as Kent's Scale of Ascending Potencies is a useful means of regulating the dosage of homeopathic remedies.[10] In acute otitis media, the chosen remedy is given once every hour to four hours depending upon the severity of the child's condition. The remedy is continued until progress stalls. At this point, the initial remedy is discounted and replaced by the same remedy at the next higher potency. Thus, if *Pulsatilla* 12x worked initially, but symptoms reappeared after 36 to 48 hours, *Pulsatilla* 30x would be given next. Obviously, if there is no improvement in the child's condition within this period, the wrong remedy was chosen. In this situation, a reevaluation of the case is required.

Constitutional care often requires the prescription of higher potencies (200x to 1M)* since they are deeper-acting. These dosages are given infrequently. Often, the prescriber gives one dose of the high-potency remedy, and observes progress for the next three to eight weeks before prescribing again.

Remedies Used in Chronic Otitis Media and Otitis Media With Effusion

The following remedies are listed in alphabetical order for easy reference. This is not an order of their frequency of use in otitis media. Also, this is an abbreviated materia medica. It may be necessary to consult a complete materia medica. For remedies used in acute otitis media and otitis media without effusion, refer to chapter 6.

It is important to note that a child need not display all the symptoms of a medicine in order for that medicine to be effective.

Baryta carbonica

In this child, the tonsils are almost always swollen. When colds occur, which they do frequently, they usually begin as a sore throat. Cold air affects his tonsils adversely. When otorrhea occurs, it is often bloody. This child is physically shorter than other children his age and is often described as dwarfish. He is slow to develop and is usually behind his peers in learning to walk and talk, in gaining weight, and in most other areas.[11] If he tries to exert himself, he becomes very tired and weak to the point of feeling exhausted. This child has poor posture, commonly a lumbar lordosis, coupled with a hard, distended abdomen. He tends to salivate heavily.

Emotionally, the *Baryta carb* child is touchy and irritable. He does not like to be interfered with. There is a fear of being left alone, going out of doors, or being around strangers. Excessive shyness is a characteristic of the *Baryta carb* child. Nightmares are common.

Mentally, this child is inattentive, forgetful, and has a short atten-

---

*Only an experienced homeopath should consider prescribing potencies in this range.

tion span. He may play with an object for one moment, then drop it and move on to something else. If he learns a new task or verse, he may forget it within a few hours or by the next day. He is often not sure he is doing the right thing.

This is one of the grand remedies for use in children with Down syndrome (although its use is by no means restricted to such children).

Symptoms are worse: from washing, bathing, and lying down.

Symptoms are better: from open air.

Calcarea carbonica

Calcarea is commonly used as a constitutional medicine. There is a tendency toward collections of fluid in various parts of the body including the middle ear. There is a thick, muco-purulent discharge from the middle ear, enlarged lymph nodes, and swollen tonsils. Recurrent infections and excessive production of mucus in the respiratory tract are important physical signs.

The *Calcarea* child is thirsty and prefers cold drinks. He craves indigestible things to eat such as chalk, pencils, or dirt. He also craves salt, eggs, raw potatoes, and sweets. Milk disagrees with him. There is usually a definite dislike of hot food, with a craving for cold things like ice cream.

Physically, the child in need of *Calcarea* is soft, plump, fair-skinned, and lethargic. He is often overweight. He is weak, easily tired, and content to just sit around doing nothing. The *Calcarea* child is sluggish in movement and does poorly at games. The slightest exertion causes him to sweat. He may have head sweats during sleep. Mentally, this child is slow and may have difficulty in school. He often lacks the motivation to persevere in mental tasks. Fearfulness and apprehension are common *Calcarea* traits. After *Baryta carb*, this is the most commonly indicated remedy for children with Down syndrome (although its use is by no means restricted to such children).

While the above signs accurately describe the *Calcarea* child, recognize that this medicine is used commonly for various complaints of infancy.

Symptoms are worse: from cold, damp weather, and mental or physical exertion.

Symptoms are better: from dry weather, lying down on the painful side, and warmth.

Calcarea sulphuricum

The *Calcarea sulph* child typically displays mucus discharges that are yellow, thick, and lumpy. There is often a discharge of yellow matter from the eyes. Otorrhea is thick, muco-purulent, and bloody. Pimples and pustules on the face are not uncommon. The soles of the feet burn and itch. There are no marked emotional signs that indicate *Calcarea sulph*.

Capsicum

This remedy is useful when the inflammation has spread to the mastoid process and there is chronic suppuration of the tympanic membrane, accompanied by bursting headache and chilliness. There are burning and stinging pains in the ear, which extend to the throat. There is great swelling and pain behind ears. This remedy is also useful in the perforation of the membrane with purulent discharge. The ear is tender to touch.[12] When coughing occurs, painful symptoms are often experienced in distant parts of the body such as the legs or ears. There is much thirst, but drinking causes this child to shiver.

This remedy suits plethoric, sluggish, cold, and weak children with diminished vital heat.

Symptoms are worse: from uncovering, drafts, and open air.

Symptoms are better: while eating and from heat.

Carbo vegetabilis

The typical *Carbo* child is sluggish, overweight, and lazy. He seems to have never fully recovered from the effects of some previous illness. The body is almost bluish and is icy-cold. The face is pale. Emotionally he fears the dark. Nosebleeds are common.

Any overindulgence causes headaches. The child experiences contractive pain in the abdomen. Eructations, heaviness, and fullness are characteristic digestive signs. Digestion is slow. The child is averse to milk, meat, and fat. He is distressed by the simplest foods. This remedy is sometimes used for children with intestinal colic. The abdomen is often greatly distended. A dry cough with hoarseness that worsens in the evening accompanies wheezing with rattling of mucus in the chest. This child is cold from the knees down to the feet. The skin is a cold blue, but perspiration is hot.

Symptoms are worse: from cold, fat food, butter, milk, warm damp weather, open air, and in evening.

Symptoms are better: from eructation and fanning.

Hepar sulphuricum

Hepar sulph is generally not used in the early stages of an earache. It is used when symptoms have progressed and pus has formed in the middle ear. There is frequently a nasal discharge that is at first watery, then becomes thick, yellow, and offensive. There is intense throbbing pain in the ear, accompanied by diminished hearing. These children are irritable and sensitive. Like the *Chamomilla* child, the *Hepar* child is cross and easily angered. They can be provoked to a tantrum with little effort. A hallmark of the *Hepar* child is over-sensitivity to touch, cold, and pain. The cold sensitivity may be so great that even a hand or foot exposed from beneath the covers results in aggravation of symptoms.

Symptoms are worse: from dry cold winds, cold foods, touch, pressure, night, exertion, or the slightest draft.

Symptoms are better: from warmth, extra clothing or covers, humidity, hot applications, and after eating.

Hydrastis

Hydrastis has an especially strong action on the mucous membranes. This remedy is characterized by secretions that are thick, yellow-ish, and ropy regardless of which area of the body is involved. There is roaring in the ears, hearing loss, and a chronic muco-purulent discharge. Eustachian catarrh is common. There is a thick mucus secretion that runs from the nasopharynx down the back of the throat. Meanwhile, a watery secretion is discharged through the nares. This child is weak, has poor digestion, and suffers from constipation. There may be a dry, harsh cough that progresses to bronchial catarrh in later stages.

Kali bichromicum

Children in need of this remedy typically have a tough, stringy, viscous discharge from the mucous membranes. What distinguishes the discharge of *Kali bic* is its sticky, gluey quality. Whether the discharge is from the nose, ears, or lungs, it has this distinctive quality.

Another characteristic of this remedy is pains that migrate quickly. The pain may be in one area, then move to another. At another point the pain may be gone. This child is usually worse in the morning. From 2 A.M. to 3 A.M., most symptoms are aggravated. He is better from heat, but hot weather makes him worse. *Kali bic* should never be used when there is fever.

Symptoms are worse: from hot weather, undressing, cold, from 2 A.M. TO 3 A.M., and in the morning.

Symptoms are better: from warmth.

Lycopodium

A characteristic of this remedy is symptoms that are on or begin on the right side. There may be a humming and roaring sensation in the ear with diminished hearing. A thick, yellow, offensive discharge is common. The nose is stopped up. There is often a viscous and offensive perspiration, especially on the feet and axillae. *Lycopodium* is especially indicated in the child with digestive complaints such as gas and bloating. Digestion is poor and irregular. Eating the tiniest amount causes fullness. The child is thin and weak. He often has cold hands and feet. Symptoms are aggravated between 4 to 8 P.M. or from 4 P.M. to midnight.

The *Lycopodium* child is fearful, apprehensive, and afraid to be alone. Sometimes the child wants to be alone, but needs to have someone nearby or in the next room. He is averse to taking on new things. He can be headstrong and scornful when sick. Fright, anger, or embarrassment may likely bring on illness. This is a remedy that may be used at any stage of an earache.

Symptoms are worse: from lying on the right side, heat or a warm room, hot air, cold food or drink, eating, and from 4 P.M. to 8 P.M.

Symptoms are better: from warm food and drink, being uncovered, cool or open air, motion, and after midnight.

Mercurius

Mercurius is indicated when there is pus formation and is often used in more chronic cases of otitis media. The nasal discharge is yellow-green and offensive (as are all body secretions in these children). There is profuse, offensive perspiration. Lymph nodes are chronically swollen. Tonsils are swollen and may be covered with pockets of pus and open sores. The gums are soft, swollen, and bleed easily. There is great thirst. The skin is almost constantly moist. If the skin is consistently dry, *Mercurius* is not the remedy. Increased salivation, bad breath, and puffiness of the tongue are general *Mercurius* symptoms.

The child in need of *Mercurius* is often described as a human "thermometer" because she is acutely sensitive to heat, cold, and nearly all environmental influences. The *Mercurius* child is weak and may tire at the slightest exertion. There is sometimes muscular trembling. This child seems to display a loss of will-power. She is agitated, hurried, impulsive, and has difficulty concentrating.

Symptoms are worse: from damp, cold, rainy weather, heat, sweating, motion, exertion, open air, lying on the right side, at night, and in a warm bed or warm room.

Symptoms are better: in moderate temperatures.

Natrum muriaticum

Natrum mur is indicated when there is great weakness and weariness. The mental signs are perhaps the most useful in this child because emotional events are often what precipitates illness in him. This is the child who becomes ill when there is fighting between parents, a public scolding, or loss of a family member or anyone close to him. If he is brought to anger, he may become ill because he is easily angered, but does not freely express his feelings. The *Natrum mur* child is irritable and is infuriated by seemingly trivial things. He rarely cries in public, but may cry alone. Any attempts to console him may be met with anger. He is oversensitive to stimulus and easily startled.

The child awakens with much sneezing. Heavy nasal discharge, described as having a raw egg-white appearance, is present. Small eruptions or vesicles form around the lips. The lips and corners of the mouth are dry, ulcerated, and cracked. A crack in the middle of the lower lip is sometimes seen.

Symptoms are worse: from noise, consolation, lying down, heat, talking, and in a warm room.

Symptoms are better: from cold bathing, lying on right side, going without regular meals, and in open air.

Psorinum

The child in need of *Psorinum* is extremely sensitive to cold. He wants his head kept warm and wants warm clothing even in summer. The child catches cold easily. Weakness persists long after recovery. All body secretions have an offensive smell. Emotionally, this child is melancholy with feelings of hopelessness and despair. There are frequently red, raw, oozing scabs around the ears that release an offensive discharge. This is accompanied by intense itching. The face also may contain skin eruptions. There is chronic, offensive otorrhea of a brownish color. There is great swelling of the tonsils with painful swallowing.

The *Psorinum* child is always hungry and desires to eat in the middle of the night. He experiences hay fever, which returns irregularly every year. The hallmark of this child is problems with the skin. There is intolerable itching that often keeps him awake at night. Eruptions occur on the scalp and at the bends of joints. Exertion causes urticaria.

Symptoms are worse: from changes of weather, cold, and the slightest draft.

Symptoms are better: from heat, warm clothing, and in summer.

Pulsatilla

Pulsatilla is not commonly indicated in chronic otitis media. However, when the constitutional picture is that of *Pulsatilla*, the healing response can be dramatic even in chronic otitis media. *Pulsatilla* is suitable for almost all types of ear pain. The child who needs *Pulsatilla* is gentle, weepy, sensitive, and loves to be held. He desires attention and is easily consoled by a sympathetic response. The *Pulsatilla* child is sometimes described as moody because he can be happy one moment and profoundly sad the next. He often feels sorry for himself and laments his plight during illness.

The cheeks are pale. He feels better when in open, fresh air. There is a thick, bland, yellowish-green nasal discharge. The eardrum is swollen and red, with fluid. If the ear is draining, the discharge is usually thick and yellowish-green. The ear is swollen, red, and hot, and there is deep itching in it. The pain often goes through the whole side of the face. There may be a stopped sensation in the ear. A dry or loose cough can be present. Symptoms often come on gradually and frequently follow a cold. The child may be feverish, but show a surprising absence of thirst.

Symptoms are worse: from heat, lying down, exertion, after eating, toward evening, and in a warm room.

Symptoms are better: with motion, cold applications, cold food and drink, and in open air.

Silica

According to Randall Neustaedter, C.A., *Silica* is the most frequently indicated constitutional remedy for chronic otitis media. He reports that, of 21 cases of chronic or recurrent otitis media, 43 percent responded favorably to treatment with *Silica*.[13] The child in need of *Silica* is likely to experience discharge from the ear. He is sensitive and anxious. *Silica* is often indicated when a cold or bronchial condition is long-standing or slow to respond. Symptoms are severe. There is often roaring in the ears, and the child is sensitive to noise. The *Silica* child is cold, chilly, and wants plenty of warm clothing. He hates drafts, and his hands and feet are icy cold. There is offensive sweat on the hands, feet, and axillae. *Silica* is the remedy most often required when there is pain behind the ear on the mastoid process. (See also *Hepar sulph*) Repair of the tympanic membrane can more often be achieved with Silica than with any other remedy.[14]

Emotionally this child is yielding, faint-hearted, and anxious. He is nervous, excitable, and sensitive, but can be obstinate. The *Silica* child tends to be weak and is easily exhausted.

Symptoms are worse: from cold, open air, winter, damp weather, cold food or drink, lying on the painful side, eating, and in morning.

Symptoms are better: from warmth.

Sulphur

Sulphur is especially indicated when there is an extensive history of antibiotic use. It has an exceptional ability to arouse the bodily defenses when they have been suppressed due to long-standing illness or drugs. The mucous membranes are characteristically hot, dry, and red. The mouth and lips may burn. There may be redness around the anus with itching. Most *Sulphur* children have constipation, although they may sometimes awaken with diarrhea. The *Sulphur* child urinates copious amounts of colorless urine. There is frequent urination with enuresis. Burning of the hands, soles of the feet, and top of the head is common.

Breathing is sometimes difficult, and the child feels better when the window is open or when out of doors. The skin is dry, scaly, and unhealthy. Every injury tends to open and become infected. The skin itches and burns. Scratching or bathing irritates the skin immensely, but bathing aggravates nearly all symptoms. All body discharges are offensive, especially perspiration.

The *Sulphur* child is quite thirsty and drinks much liquid, although milk causes digestive upset. He is very weak and faint around 11 A.M. and must have something to eat. The *Sulphur* child has a well-developed appetite with very definite taste preferences. Yet, he becomes sluggish and tired after meals. Cold weather and fresh air invigorate the *Sulphur* child. Emotionally, the child is self-centered and demanding. He is often overconcerned with possessions and may take great pride in his toys, which he often hoards.

Symptoms are worse: from bathing, washing, cold air, warmth, standing, scratching, at 11 A.M., and on the left side.

Symptoms are better: from dry, warm weather; lying on right side, open air, and warm drinks.

Tellurium

Tellurium is not a common remedy in otitis media, but when the constitutional picture matches, it can be invaluable. There is eczema behind the ear and middle ear catarrh that may drain outward. Otorrhea is acrid, often described as smelling like "fish-pickle." It is watery, but frequently excoriating (tending to abrade the surrounding skin). There is intense itching, swelling, and throbbing in the ear canal. The child in need of *Tellurium* has a very sensitive back. Pain usually runs from the seventh cervical vertebra to the fifth thoracic. These children are very sensitive to touch. Even the friction of clothing may be bothersome. There may be sacral and sciatic pains.

This remedy is characterized by circular patches (like ringworm) on the skin, accompanied by itching. Emotionally the child is neglectful and forgetful. The action of this remedy may take long to develop.

Symptoms are worse: from coughing, laughing, touch, lying on the painful side, while at rest at night, and in cold weather.

Symptoms are better: The coryza, lachrymation, and hoarseness are better in open air.

Manipulation

When otitis media is due to dysfunctional mechanics in the upper cervical spine, manual manipulation of the affected vertebrae should be considered an essential part of treatment. According to Gutmann, "... in this syndrome [occipito-atlanto-axial joint dysfunction] the success of adjustment over shadows every other type of treatment, especially the pharmaceutical approach...."[15]

Spinal Problems

A. History: The history will frequently, but not always, contain incidences of trauma to the head or neck.

   1. Trauma (macrotrauma or microtrauma)

      a. Birth

         —Vacuum extraction

         —Forceps

         —Cesarean section

         —Prolonged or difficult vaginal delivery

         —Normal birth*

         —First child

      b. Other injuries

         —Rough play with peers

         —Falls from changing table, bed, down stairs, etc.

         —Overzealous play by parents (throwing or spinning the child)

         —Physical abuse by caregiver

   2. General

      The following generalized signs have been found to be associated with upper cervical biomechanical dysfunction. Some of these signs may indicate more serious disease, so the physician should proceed with the full spectrum of diagnostic possibilities in mind.

         —Lowered resistance to infection of the ear, nose, and throat

         —Conjunctivitis

         —Sleeping difficulty

         —Neck pain, stiffness, or rigidity

---

*Strong uterine contractions may contribute to musculoskeletal injury even during a delivery which is considered normal or uneventful.

—Headaches

—Torticollis (especially infantile)

—Seizures

—Vomiting

—Hyperactivity

—Morphological deformations of the bony skeleton

—Intestinal colic

B. Examination

   1. Palpation

      a. Motion palpation of the occipito-atlanto-axial complex

      —Observe for abnormal relational movement of the vertebrae on flexion, extension, right and left rotation, and lateral flexion.

      b. Static palpation of the occipito-atlanto-axial complex

      c. Palpation of soft tissue

      —Note areas of swelling, muscle spasm and rigidity, areas of muscle hypotonicity, heat, and tenderness.

      —Note "feel" and tenderness of local acupoints.

   2. Radiographic

      a. X-ray analysis is used by some to establish proper line of drive and contact, not to establish mechanical relationships.

      b. In cases of trauma, X-ray should be considered to rule out fracture, dislocation, instability of atlanto-axial ligament, basilar invagination, etc.

      c. There is a high incidence of atlanto-axial instability in children with Down syndrome due to laxity of the transverse atlantal ligament, or anomalous axis formation. Since this is a high-risk group for otitis media, it is important to know that upper cervical manipulation in these children can result in fatal consequences. For a review of the chiropractic evaluation and management of the Down syndrome child refer to "A Chiropractic Perspective in Atlantoaxial Instability in Down's Syndrome."[16]

—Note that when the initial bout of otitis media begins early in life, for example at 0–5 months, functional problems of the cervical spine should be considered.

C. Mechanical Findings

In otitis media, a number of possible structural relationships may occur in the cervical spine. The most common biomechanical contributor to otitis media is atlanto-occipital dysfunction (or subluxation).

1. Occiput. It is more common to find the side of subluxation on the same side as the middle ear involvement. However, this does not always occur. Bilateral otitis media often occurs with bilateral occipital involvement.

    a. Anterior right, left, or bilateral

    b. Posterior right, left, or bilateral

    c. Lateral right or left

2. 1st Cervical (C1, also known as the atlas). Subluxation of C1 occurs frequently in otitis media. Like occipital involvement, C1 involvement is commonly on the same side as the middle ear problem. Bilateral otitis media often occurs with bilateral C1 involvement.

    a. Anterior right, left, or bilateral

    b. Posterior right, left, or bilateral

    c. Lateral right or left

3. 2nd Cervical (C2, also known as the axis). Subluxation of C2 is present less frequently in otitis media than is subluxation of C1 or occiput. When this occurs, it is usually posterior or lateral. Anteriority is less common, but does occur.

    a. Anterior right, left, or bilateral

    b. Posterior right, left, or bilateral

    c. Lateral right or left

  4. Thoracic mobilization may be indicated, especially when there is respiratory congestion. Thoracic mobilization has been shown to enhance immune function.

In acute otitis media, if biomechanical involvement is a chief contributor, symptoms should abate within 24 hours following treatment. If they do not, other factors are responsible. Even when biomechanical problems are believed to be present in acute otitis media, it is necessary to address dietary and nutritional factors as well. Homeopathic care, acupuncture, and allergy management are vital adjuncts that should be considered in the overall management. It is my opinion that only a small percentage of children with otitis media due to biomechanical problems require manipulation alone. The majority of cases require adjunctive care as well.

In chronic otitis media, manipulation can only be considered one aspect of the treatment plan. In these children, the degree of constitutional weakness and middle ear inflammation is significant. The overall strategy must involve assessment and management of diet, food allergy, and nutrition. I've found that homeopathic medicine, acupuncture, and botanical medicine are the most successful means of restoring a child with constitutional weakness to optimum health. Children with acute or chronic otitis media may require antibiotic intervention at various stages. Under these circumstances, it is still important to manage biomechanical problems.

The above discussion only represents suggestions. The clinician should conduct a customary physical examination to determine the precise state of cervical biomechanics. It is assumed that those engaging in manipulative therapy have had prior professional training in manipulation. Those without training should not attempt manipulation of the cervical spine, especially in children.

Temperomandibular Joint Problems

Temperomandibular joint (TMJ) dysfunction, while not proven to be a cause of recurrent otitis media in children, is a suspected contributor. In adults, TMJ dysfunction often results in symptoms of ear pain, fullness of the ear, and sometimes hearing deficit.

Unfortunately, the causes or TMJ problems are many and management is complex. Bruxism* is often a cause of TMJ dysfunction in children (although it can be a result of TMJ dysfunction as well). Bruxism can be brought on by parasites, allergies, emotional stress, or other factors. TMJ problems also can develop in children who are bottlefed from infancy. The nutritional inadequacy of formula, coupled with the reduced sucking associated with bottlefeeding results in potential malformation of the jaw, cranial bones, and bite. There are presently no universally accepted means of diagnosis and treatment of TMJ dysfunction.

Articular Strains of the Cranium

Trauma at birth contributes to articular strains in the newborn cranium that persist into childhood unless corrective steps are taken. Normal pelvic forces cause great shifting of the cranial bones as the child emerges from the birth canal. When forceps are used, the resulting strains can be significant.

When examining the newborn, infant, toddler, or older child with otitis media, facial symmetry should be considered. Careful observation often reveals asymmetry in the maxillae, zygomatic arches, temporal bones, parietal bones, and other less conspicuous cranial structures. Cranial asymmetry suggests fixation of the sutures at some location. In some children with otitis media, it may be necessary to correct this fixation before progress can occur.

The role of cranial manipulation in managing otitis media is not clearly established. However, numerous clinical accounts suggest that it can be of great value.

---

*Bruxism is defined as grinding of the teeth, especially during sleep.

Acupuncture

Material in this section (except where noted) was reprinted from *The Treatment of Children by Acupuncture,* by Julian Scott, Ph.D., published by the Journal of Chinese Medicine. (Please note that the original manuscript was formatted in a way that might provide added meaning.) Dr. Scott's book is the definitive work on pediatric acupuncture, and I highly recommend it for anyone who treats children. The format is clear and concise.

This section contains a very specialized vocabulary which may seem technical to those unfamiliar with acupuncture. However, since this chapter is intended for practitioners I have assumed prior knowledge of terms. For more information on acupuncture see the suggested reading section of the appendices.

* * *

Otitis media is common among children of all ages, and those who are prone may have repeated attacks. It causes great distress, and for many conditions (especially viral in origin), there is no treatment in Western medicine. Acupuncture offers a cure both in the acute phase and as a preventive against repeated attacks. In Western medicine, otitis is always regarded as being due to external attack of viral or bacterial origin. In Chinese medicine, some conditions are regarded as due to external pathogenic wind and others as due to internal heat flaring up in the liver channel.

This approach helps to explain why some children are more prone to attacks than others. If internal heat (either Ji-heat or liver heat) already exists, then it is easy for external pathogenic factors to enter. The cause of heat in very young children is Ji-blockage, while in children of seven years and above, the heat may be due to emotional causes, especially emotional tension generated by trying to please over-ambitious parents.

Regarding external pathogenic factors, it is easy for any upper respiratory tract infection to spread to the ears and cause otitis. Once established, it may return frequently in the syndrome of 'pathogenic factor remaining.' Another common cause is water in the ear from too much swimming. This is especially common among children who swim as a spare-time activity in the evening and who are thus prone to being over-tired.

As far as the differentiation of syndromes is concerned, the main distinctions presented here are as follows:

i) Non-purulent, or catarrhal, as opposed to purulent. The catarrhal type often has little or no discharge from the ear or nose, and if there is any discharge it is clear and watery. By contrast, the purulent type always has a thick yellow discharge, often foul-smelling. The purulent type is basically similar to the catarrhal, but it has the additional complication of damp building up in the body.

ii) Acute as opposed to chronic. Here chronic means more or less continuous earache, usually with discharge. Chronic otitis may have periods of acute attack.

iii) External cause as opposed to internal. The external cause is wind or damp obstructing the ear cavities, and the internal cause is liver-heat or damp heat in the liver entering the channel and causing obstruction. In practice, many acute attacks have both an internal and an external factor. It is then for the practitioner to decide on the emphasis of treatment.

In carrying out a diagnosis on a child with an acute attack or with recurrent attacks, the ear area should be palpated for tenderness and for swollen glands. The otoscope is useful in determining the severity of the condition and in assessing the progress of treatment.

Etiology and Pathology

A. Acute catarrhal

1. Etiology

External pathogenic wind, either in the form of an infection which spreads to the ear or cold wind blowing on the ear; or damp pathogenic factor from damp weather or too much swimming; or heat which affects the liver and gall bladder channels.

2. Pathology

The ear cavity receives jing from the kidneys and yang qi from the channels. Jing and yang together allow hearing to take place. If there is invasion of pathogenic heat, wind, or damp, it can block the qi and cause obstruction. The obstruction enters the cavities, giving rise to deafness and a distending or bursting sensation in the ear.

The most common cause is external pathogenic wind which blocks up the ear cavities so that the inside and outside become unregulated. The other main cause is liver and gall bladder oppressed heat which enters the channels and rises up to the ear cavities, causing the qi to knot and the jing-luo to become stuck and obstructed, giving rise to otitis media.

B. Acute Purulent

1. Etiology

Invasion of external pathogenic wind-heat poison, often originating in the respiratory tract and rising up to the ear due to excessively spicy, heating, or damp-producing foods; or Ji-heat causing heat and damp in the liver and gall bladder channels.

2. Pathology

The zheng-qi cannot resist the pathogenic factor of wind-heat/damp-poison. The pathogenic factor passes to the eardrum and then to the middle ear, where it causes stagnation of fluid. The stagnant fluid transforms to pus which is discharged through the external ear. Alternatively, liver and gall bladder damp-heat enters the channels and rises up, penetrating the ear cavities where it collects and transforms into pus.

C. Chronic catarrhal

1. Etiology

The result of acute otitis media which is not cured or only partially cured (pathogenic factor remaining), or the body is feeble and weak from overwork or long-term disease.

Acute

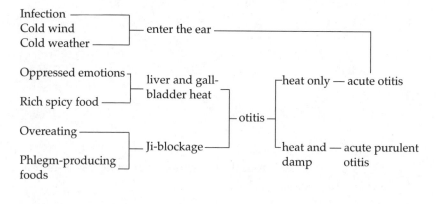

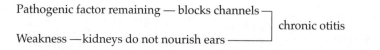

Otitis media

2. Pathology

The pathogenic factor remains and is not cleared, blocking up the ear cavities so that the qi and blood are stuck and obstructed; or the body is weak and the liver and kidney jing are insufficient; or the spleen qi is xu and weak, so that the jing is without the support necessary to send it up. The ear cavity is then without nourishment.

Clinical Manifestations and Differentiation of Syndromes

A. Acute catarrhal

1. Pathogenic wind enters the cavities

—Ear stuffed up, hearing power reduced

—Tinnitus

—Mild ear pain

—Ear drum bleeding slightly

—Occasional upper respiratory tract infection

—Dislikes cold

—Fever

—Headache

—Nasal discharge

Pulse: floating

Treatment principle: Expel wind and clear heat, regulate the ear cavity, and drain damp.

2. Liver and gall bladder oppressed heat

—Inner ear distended and full, bleeding from eardrum, fluid in ear passage

—Dizziness

—Headache with swollen feeling, pressure, and bursting sensation

—Buzzing in ears, hearing power reduced

Tongue: body red

Tongue coat: yellow

Pulse: wiry or slippery, rapid

Treatment principle: Clear liver and gall bladder heat, resolve damp, and regulate the ear cavity.

B. Acute purulent

1. Wind-heat at the superficial level

Before the purulent stage, there are the symptoms and signs characteristic of wind-heat:

—Uncomfortable body

—Dislikes wind

—Chills and maybe fevers

—Headache

followed by:

—Earache and ear pain

—Hearing power reduced

—Discharge of pus and blood from the ear; pus often pale or milky

Tongue coat: thin

Pulse: floating, rapid

Treatment principle: Expel wind and relieve the exterior, clear heat, and resolve poison.

2. Liver and gall bladder damp-heat

—Inflammation that does not subside

—Headache

—Ear region swollen and painful; eardrum discharges blood; mastoid process mildly painful; outer and middle ear filled with yellow pus

—Stools dry

—May be vomiting and twitching

Tongue coat: greasy, yellow

Tongue body: red

Pulse: wiry, slippery

Treatment principle: Clear heat and bring down damp, resolve poison, reduce swelling, stop pain.

C. Chronic catarrhal

General:

—Tinnitus

—Deafness

—Middle ear full and packed

—Examination shows white distended eardrum.

1. Pathogenic factor remaining

—Distending and bursting sensation in the middle ear

—The ear feels blocked. On examination one eardrum may be seen to be bleeding slightly or discharging clear fluid.

—May have nose bleed

—May have nose and throat inflammation

—May have swollen glands behind the ear and in the neck

—May have recurrent attacks of acute catarrhal otitis

Pulse: slow or moderate, slippery

Treatment principle: Move qi and disperse blockage, circulate blood, and expel the pathogenic factor.

2a. Liver and kidney insufficient

—Dizziness

—Sticky fluid on the eardrum

—May have sore back

Tongue: tip of tongue red

Pulse: fine, rapid

Treatment principle: Support and reinforce liver and kidney; move and regulate the cavities.

2b. Spleen-qi xu and weak

—Inner ear swollen and bursting

—Eardrum grey-white in color

—Patient comparatively lazy and without strength

—Mouth and lips pale

—Easily discouraged

—Poor appetite

Tongue body: pale

Pulse: fine, weak

Treatment principle: Tonify the spleen and bring up jing; move the ear cavity, and resolve damp.

Treatment

Main Points

The ear is encircled by the hand shaoyang (sanjiao) channel, and a secondary channel passes through the ear from Fengchi GB-20. Consequently the main points to use are on the hand and foot shaoyang channels:

Fengchi GB-20 To expel wind and regulate the liver and gall bladder

Yifeng SJ-17 To expel wind and benefit the ear

Tinghui GB-2 Local point

Waiguan SJ-5 To expel wind and regulate the sanjiao channel

Zulinqi GB-41 To regulate the liver and gall bladder

Method: Fengchi GB-20 is needled slightly laterally, to direct the sensation to the ear. Yifeng SJ-17 is needled to a depth of 1 cun. Tinghui GB-2 may be needled to a depth of 1½ cun, but in shi conditions it is usually sufficient to needle to a depth of ½ cun. The sensation should radiate to the inner ear and is usually rather painful. Waiguan SJ-5 and Zulinqi GB-41 are needled to a depth of ½ to 1 cun, and the sensation should go upwards along the limb, towards the head.

According to differentiation of syndromes

A. Acute catarrhal

   1. Pathogenic wind enters the cavities.

     Provided there are no signs of heat, moxa may be used on Yifeng SJ-17. This will bring quick relief. In addition, add:

        Hegu LI-4   To clear wind

     Prognosis: In babies and young children, one treatment using distal points alone is often enough. The children break out into a sweat, then fall asleep and are cured. Older children may require three treatments (given in one day). If this does not cure the condition, it usually means that it is a different syndrome.

2. Liver and gall bladder oppressed heat

The main points given above are usually sufficient. Alternative points are:

Zhongzhu SJ-3   In place of Waiguan SJ-5

Qiuxu GB-40   In place of Zulinqi GB-41

Prognosis: This condition is common among older children and may take several treatments (three to five) to cure. In cases of very acute pain, give treatment twice or even three times daily. After that, once a day.

B. Acute purulent

1. Pathogenic wind-heat

In addition to the main points, the following points will be of use:

Hegu LI-4   These three points used together
Dazhui Du-14   are very effective in clearing
Quchi LI-11   pathogenic wind-heat.

If there is constipation, a purge should be administered.

Prognosis: One or two treatments are usually sufficient, though it may take more in stubborn cases.

2. Liver and gall bladder damp-heat

In addition to the main points, the following points may be used:

Yinlingquan SP-9   To clear damp-heat

Yanglingquan GB-34   To transform damp in shao yang channel

Zhangmen LIV-13   To transform damp

Method: Four to five points are selected on the affected side. Treat once a day or twice a day in very young children.

Prognosis: This is usually rather slow to change, and there may be no appreciable result until after the third treatment. Usually eight to ten treatments are sufficient.

C. Chronic catarrhal

1. Pathogenic factor remaining

In addition to the main points, the following may be of service:

Bailao (extra)	2 cun superior to Dazhui DU-14, one cun lateral to the spine. To clear remaining pathogenic factors.
Ganshu BL-18	To regulate the liver and gall bladder, and move blood and qi.
Pishu BL-20	To regulate the spleen, move blood and qi, and resolve damp.

Method: Needle or moxa may be used on these points.

Prognosis: To clear the body completely of the pathogenic factor may take ten to twenty treatments.

2a. Liver and kidney insufficient

Local points are not usually of much service, except in cases of acute pain, and even then their effect is short-term.

Distal points should be used, e.g.:

Waiguan SJ-5	These points all have
Yanglingquan GB-34	the function of
Ganshu BL-18	tonifying the liver and
Shenshu BL-23	kidney yin.
Taichong LIV-3	
Taixi KI-3	

Prognosis: This condition is uncommon in children, except after febrile disease, when a few treatments will suffice, provided that the child is eating normally. If the condition occurs without a history of febrile disease, it is essential to discover the cause for the yin-xu condition.

2b. Spleen-qi xu and weak

Again, local points are not usually of much service. Preferable points are:

Waiguan SJ-5	To move qi in the ear
Yanglingquan GB-34	To move qi in the ear
Zusanli ST-36	To tonify the spleen and resolve damp
Sanyinjiao SP-6	To tonify the spleen and resolve damp
Zhongwan REN-12	To tonify the spleen and resolve damp
Hegu LI-4	To tonify the spleen and resolve damp
Pishu BL-20	To tonify the spleen and resolve damp

In babies, Si feng (extra) may be used [located on the palmar surface, in the transverse creases of the proximal interphalangeal joints of the index, middle, ring, and little fingers].

Moxa may be used, especially on the abdominal and back points.

Method: Treat twice or three times a week.

Prognosis: Three to five treatments are usually enough, provided that the patient can rest.

Notes

1. It is often difficult to distinguish between external attack of pathogenic wind, and liver and gall bladder heat conditions, since if there is mental irritation leading to a mild build-up of heat, the child is more susceptible to wind conditions.

2. Repeated treatment with antibiotics can lead to a build-up of damp.

3. In all otitis, the patient should avoid red meat and spicy, fried, and other heating foods. If dampness is present, they should also avoid eggs, cheese, milk, peanuts, and sugar. [Damp conditions are frequently more slow to respond.]

* * *

Discharge as a Diagnostic Indicator

Nasal discharge or otorrhea are commonly found in children with otitis media. The color of this discharge often provides useful diagnostic information. Special consideration should be given to the consistency and color of any discharge found. The most common colors are clear, white, yellow, and green.

Discharge	Indication
Clear	Wind-cold, damp
White	Phlegm
Yellow	Heat or bacterial infection
Green	Wind or viral infection

Needle Technique

Needles should be 1/2 to 1 inch in length and of 32 gauge. They are inserted quickly into the skin, and then manipulated to the required depth to obtain *de qi*. Needle retention is unnecessary in children under 10 years of age,[17] i.e., the needles are quickly withdrawn following *de qi*. A minimum number of needles should be used in children, usually only four to six.[18]

An obstacle that must be overcome when using acupuncture with children is fear of needles. Surprisingly, children do not object to acupuncture to the degree one would expect. More commonly it is the parents who fear needles. If present, these concerns should be dealt with openly before beginning treatment. Acupuncture can be used safely and effectively in children of any age.

Other Forms of Stimulation

Some doctors feel that moxa may be used effectively with children. However, others believe that use of moxa carries a risk of disrupting the San Jiao (triple heater) channel and can have an adverse effect on thermoregulation. I suggest that only the experienced acupuncturist consider using moxa on children, especially in conditions such as otitis media.

It has become popular in China, the United States, and Europe to use various methods of electrical stimulation to treat acupoints. Generally, battery-operated devices that generate a small DC electrical current are either applied to needles inserted into acupoints, or a probe is placed on the point for direct stimulation. I recommend that such devices not be used on children. There are several good reasons for this:

- The levels of current and voltage generated by such devices are high.

- No one is yet certain of the current and voltage thresholds of a young child's body.

- Electrolysis and tissue damage is believed to occur locally when such devices are used.[19]

- Many electrical stimulation devices sold today are subjected to little or no quality control.

Until we more fully understand the direct and indirect effects of this form of stimulation, it is best to use traditional methods.

Si Feng Treatment

According to Martha Benedict, M.A., O.M.D., there is one form of acupuncture treatment that deserves special consideration in the management of otitis media in children. Dr. Benedict has a unique and valuable perspective on otitis media. She has an M.A. in audiology and speech pathology from Stanford Medical School, and was on the faculty at the University of California Medical Center as a clinician and researcher. After many years of observing the

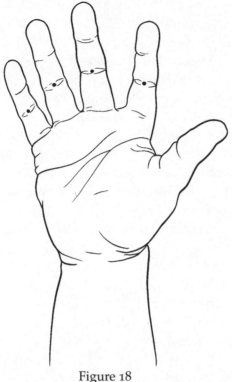

Figure 18
Location of the Si Feng Points

response (and often the lack of response) of thousands of children with otitis media to conventional care, she began her training in Chinese medicine. Her combined experiences in audiology and Chinese medicine have convinced her that most children with otitis media can be effectively treated using acupuncture and Chinese botanical medicine.

One technique used by Dr. Benedict in the management of acute and chronic otitis media is stimulation of the Si Feng points on the palmar surface of the hands. There are twelve Si Feng points. The lower Si Feng is at the metacarpophalangeal joint of the index through little finger. The middle Si Feng is at the proximal interphalangeal joint, and the upper Si Feng at the distal interphalangeal joint. (See figure 18.)

Dr. Benedict treats the middle Si Feng points by applying the technique known as bleeding.* The technique of bleeding acupoints has been used for centuries to manage febrile or inflammatory conditions. This method requires the use of a three-edged needle. When acute or chronic otitis media presents, the needle is used to prick the finger at the locations of the middle Si Feng. This will cause one or two drops of blood to be expressed.

The effects of Si Feng treatment on middle ear inflammation can be impressive. Benedict reports that improvement in the inflammatory state of the middle ear can be observed in as little as ten minutes, often while the child is still in the office. She states that acute otitis often responds fully within 24 hours. The treatment is enhanced when botanicals are used with acupuncture.

Botanical Medicine

The clinical use of botanical medicine can have a substantial impact on the underlying syndromes of both acute and chronic otitis media. Children with otitis media who require antibiotic therapy can be assisted by concurrent therapy with botanical medicine. As mentioned above, the use of botanical medicine is enhanced by the simultaneous application of acupuncture and vice versa.

In this section, I present the management of otitis media using Chinese botanical medicine. Admittedly, there are many different traditions of botanical medicine used in the world, all which have intrinsic value. However, the Chinese appear to have developed the most sophisticated and effective method of prescribing for otitis media.

Treatment of Underlying Syndrome

The practitioner of botanical medicine, like the practitioner of acupuncture, relies on a detailed examination of the patient to identify the specific syndrome involved. Once the syndrome is identified, the proper botanical formula is selected based on a few differentiating features. The differentiation of syndromes can be

---

*Only a trained acupuncturist should attempt this technique.

considered the same when using Chinese botanical medicine as when using acupuncture (although the treatment principles may differ somewhat).

Below is a presentation of the Chinese botanical formulas used to manage the various syndromes (described in Chinese medicine) encountered in otitis media.* The format is the same as that presented in the section on acupuncture. For a description of signs and symptoms associated with each syndrome, refer to the section on acupuncture titled "Clinical Manifestations and Differentiation of Syndromes."

A. Acute catarrhal

   1. Pathogenic wind enters the cavities

Formula:	Pueraria Combination	
Contains:	*Pueraria*	*Ma huang*
	Peony	*Jujube*
	Cinnamon	*Licorice*
	Ginger	

      Indications: Used in the early stages when the ear is more stuffed up but without infection.

Formula:	Bupleurum and Schizonepeta	
Contains:	*Bupleurum*	*Ginger*
	Tuhuo	*Hoelen*
	Cnidium	*Siler*
	Cherry bark	*Licorice*
	Platycodon	*Schizonepeta*

      Indications: Used in the early stages when there is slight infection.

---

*This listing of Chinese botanical formulas was compiled by Anastacia White, a professional herbalist. White is a teacher and practitioner of Chinese botanical medicine and lectures throughout the United States.[20]

2. Liver and gall bladder oppressed heat

      Formula: Minor Bupleurum

      Contains:

Bupleurum	*Pinellia*
Ginseng	*Licorice*
Ginger	*Jujube*
Scutellaria	

      Indications: Used when the patient has weak stomach and spleen with excessive dampness.

      Formula: Niu Huang Chien Tu Pien

      Contains:

Rhubarb	*Gypsum*
Scutellaria	*Ox gallstone*
Licorice	*Platycodon*
Borneol	

      Indications: Used when there are extreme heat symptoms, and the patient does not have a weak spleen.

B. Acute purulent

   1.Wind-heat at the superficial level

      Formula: Schizonepeta and Forsythia

      Contains:

Tang Kuei	*Gardenia*
Scutellaria	*Angelica*
Platycodon	*Peony*
Siler	*Mentha*
Coptis	*Forsythia*
Chih Ko	*Schizonepeta*
Bupleurum	*Rehamannia*
Phellodendron	

2. Liver and gall bladder damp-heat

      Formula: Gentiana Combination

      Contains: *Gentiana*   *Plantago*

Alisma	Tang Kuei
Akebia	Rehmannia
Gardenia	Scutellaria
Licorice	Bupleurum

C. Chronic catarrhal

1. Pathogenic factor remaining

Formula: Gleditsia Combination

Contains:
Ginseng	Atractylodes
Poria	Angelica
Cnidium	Peony
Licorice	Lonicera
Platycodon	Tang Kuei
Gleditsia	Astragalus

2a. Liver and kidney insufficient

Formula: Er Ming Zuo Ci Wan

Contains:
Rehmannia	Cornus
Dioscorea	Alisma
Mouton	Poria
Bupleurum	Magnetite Mineral

2b. Spleen-qi xu and weak

Formula: Astragalus and Platycodon
              Combination

Contains:
Ginseng	Tang Kuei
Cnidium	Licorice
Cinnamon	Siler
Astragalus	Platycodon
Angelica	Magnolia bark

To further resolve dampness add:

Formula: Citrus and Pinellia

Contains:
Citrus	Licorice
Ginger	Poria
Pinellia	

Symptomatic relief can be provided by using the Superior Sore Throat Powder Spray, which is a Chinese patent formula. The powder is applied by blowing a small amount through a straw into the ear canal. This spray can be used in conjunction with all of the above botanical formulas, with the exception of **Pueraria Combination**.

Formula: Superior Sore Throat Powder Spray

Contains: *Coptis*   *Ox gallstone*
           Borneol   *Mother of pearl*
           Licorice   *Indigo powder*
           Sophora

Besides the formulas listed above, a mixture can be prepared for use as eardrops. The combination called "The Three Yellows" is made from the oils of *Coptis*, *Phellodendron*, and *Scutellaria*. These are all "cold" herbs, which help to reduce inflammation in the middle ear. A formula known as "The Four Yellows" includes those just mentioned, with the addition of *Astragalus*, which helps eliminate pus. Both are extremely useful in managing the pain associated with otitis media.[21]

Clinical Nutrition

There is no longer any doubt that deficiency of nutrients can lead to disease. There is also no doubt that, under the right circumstances, nutritional therapy can have a substantial impact upon not only amelioration of the symptoms of disease, but the underlying causes as well. As our understanding of nutrition grows, so too do the prospects for treating otitis media with appropriate nutritional intervention.

The nutritional management of otitis media is a somewhat new area. Therefore, rather than listing specific protocols as I've done in prior sections, I will present some relevant research surrounding nutrition as it relates to controlling inflammation and enhancing immune function. This is in the hope that interested persons might expand upon the existing research on nutrition and otitis media.

Nutrition and Inflammation

In chapter 5, I briefly described how fatty acids, vitamins, and minerals affect the formation of both pro-inflammatory and anti-inflammatory prostaglandins. This understanding is important in light of discoveries that inflammatory prostaglandins, leukotrienes, and other arachidonic acid metabolites are found in substantial concentrations in the middle ear fluid of children with otitis media. Among the substances found are PGE2, 6-keto-PGF1 alpha, thromboxane B2, 5-HETE, 15-HETE, leukotriene C4, and leukotriene B4.[22]

Much pharmaceutical research has centered on developing anti-inflammatory drugs that block the formation of inflammatory prostaglandins. These are known as prostaglandin inhibitors. The elder statesmen among these drugs are cortisone and aspirin. The newer generation of PG-inhibitors include indomethacin and ibuprofen. As described earlier, besides inhibiting inflammatory prostaglandins, these drugs interfere with the normal production of most other prostaglandins. Thus, there is a great tendency to aggravate the inflammatory response, leading to more chronic health problems.

Nutritional substances, and even botanical medicines, offer an alternative to the use of NSAIDs (Non-Steroidal Anti-Inflammatory Drugs) because they block the enzymes that lead to the production of inflammatory prostaglandins, but do not adversely affect the enzymes needed for conversion of anti-inflammatory prostaglandins. There is evidence that these same nutrients also enhance the formation of the body's natural anti-inflammatory substances.

Using this knowledge, it may be possible to both control the painful symptoms of otitis media and correct the underlying inflammatory imbalance through nutritional intervention.

To understand more clearly the role of nutrients in blocking inflammation, it is necessary to first review the way in which prostaglandins are formed from fatty acids and the various enzymes that are needed for this process.

The Enzymes of Inflammation

Recall that the inflammatory response, as it relates to prostaglandins, begins with the cell membrane. The cell membrane consists of phospholipids that contain a variety of fatty acids. A principal constituent of these phospholipids is arachidonic acid. Arachidonic acid can be present in the cell membrane in large amounts depending upon the level of omega-6 fatty acids in the diet. If omega-3 fatty acids are consumed in large amounts, arachidonic acid is displaced from the phospholipids. (See EPA below.) The enzyme phospholipase A2 catalyzes the liberation of arachidonic acid from the membrane phospholipids, resulting in the creation of free arachidonic acid. This is the first step in the inflammatory pathway known as the arachidonic acid cascade.

Once free arachidonic acid is available, it undergoes further conversion by one of two pathways. Under the action of cyclo-oxygenase, arachidonic acid is converted into thromboxanes or 2-series prostaglandins. Under the action of lipoxygenase, arachidonic acid is converted into derivatives of HPETE (hydroperoxyeicosatetraenoic acid) and leukotrienes. (See figure 19.) Thromboxanes, 2-series prostaglandins, HPETE, and leukotrienes all possess a high degree of inflammation-inducing activity.

Enzymes of the Arachidonic Acid Cascade

1. Phospholipase A2—Causes arachidonic acid stored in the phospholipids of cell membranes to be released as free arachidonic acid. This is the first step toward inflammation via the arachidonic acid cascade.

2. Cyclooxygenase—Catalyzes the conversion of free arachidonic acid into prostaglandin E2, prostacyclins, and thromboxanes.

3. Lipoxygenase—Catalyzes the conversion of free arachidonic acid into leukotrienes and HPETEs (and related compounds).

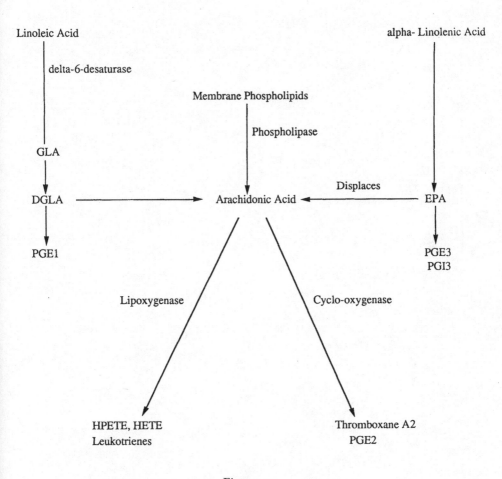

Figure 19
Prostaglandin Synthesis and the Arachidonic Acid Cascade

During conditions of excessive or prolonged inflammation, it is often desirable to reduce the substrates available for inflammation. This means balancing the intake of omega-3 and omega-6 fatty acids and in some cases, providing large amounts of certain fatty acids. It is also useful to use nutrients that block enzymes of the inflammatory pathways. Some of these are described below. (See figures 20 and 21.)

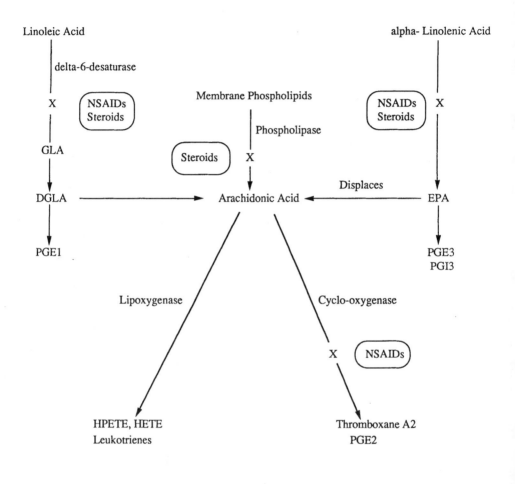

Figure 20
**The Effect of Anti-Inflammatory Drugs on Prostaglandins
and Arachidonic Acid Metabolites**

The "X" indicates where blockage of the pathway occurs. NSAID refers
to Non-Steroidal Anti-Inflammatory Drugs. Included in this are aspirin,
indomethacin, and ibuprofen. Note that NSAIDs favor the formation of
lipoxygenase products. These drugs also block the release of the more
favorable PG1 and PGE3 which is undesirable.

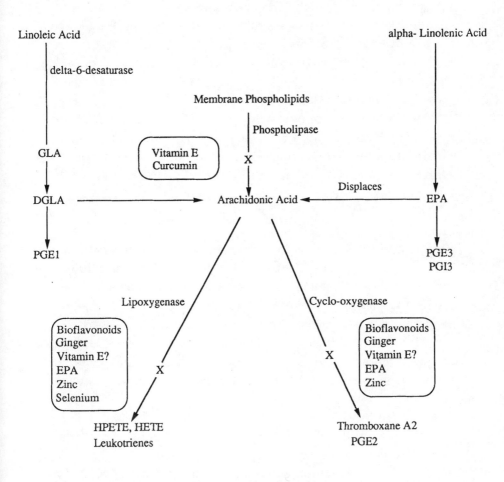

Figure 21
Nutrients That Block the Release of Inflammatory Mediators

The "X" indicates where blockage of the pathway occurs.

Vitamin C. Vitamin C is an important antioxidant nutrient that protects cells from damage by free radicals. Recently, vitamin C was found to be the "premier" antioxidant found in the body. It was shown to neutralize 100 percent of the free radicals to which it was exposed, while sparing other antioxidants.[23] Vitamin C is necessary for the proper metabolism of drugs and toxic environmental chemicals. It is also necessary for the absorption of iron. The uptake of vitamin C by leukocytes is seriously impaired when traditional anti-inflammatory drugs such as aspirin and cortisone are used. Aspirin taken daily for four days causes the leukocyte levels of ascorbic acid to fall to levels found in scurvy.[24]

Vitamin C does not appear to block the enzymes described above, but it is of vital importance in the detoxification of histamine.[25] Recall that histamine is the chemical responsible for the runny nose, watery eyes, and itchiness associated with hay fever. Histamine also plays an important role in initiating other allergy-related symptoms.

Bioflavonoids. Bioflavonoids are among the few substances that block the action of phospholipase A2, cyclo-oxygenase, and lipoxygenase.[26, 27] Therefore, they interfere with the formation of a whole range of inflammatory prostaglandins. Unlike anti-inflammatory drugs, bioflavonoids do not interfere with the enzymes needed to form PG1, PG3, and other anti-inflammatory prostaglandins. Bioflavonoids are naturally occurring substances commonly found in the same foods as vitamin C. It appears that bioflavonoids enhance the activity of vitamin C.

One example of a bioflavonoid with potent anti-inflammatory action is curcumin, found in the plant *Curcuma longa*, or turmeric. Several studies conducted in the early 1970s show that curcumin has greater anti-inflammatory action than cortisone or NSAIDs. This is, in part, due to its indirect inhibitory effect on phospholipase A2.[28, 29, 30] Curcumin is a potent scavenger of free radicals and may prevent lipid peroxidation more efficiently than beta-carotene and alpha-tocopherol. The substance has thus far been shown to produce no side effects.[31]

Quercitin, another powerful bioflavonoid, is a lipoxygenase inhibitor.[32] The use of quercitin therapeutically prevents the formation of leukotrienes, thereby reducing the symptoms of inflammation.[33] Quercitin also reduces the release of histamine and the IgE-mediated allergic response to food and environmental allergens.[34]

Ginger. Substances derived from the plant *Zingiber officinale* have an inhibitory effect on the enzymes lipoxygenase and cyclo-oxygenase, thus preventing the formation of HPETEs, leukotrienes, thromboxanes, and PG2s.[35] Ginger is among the eight herbs contained in the Japanese formula *Sairei-to*. Recall that this formula was tested for its efficacy in treating otitis media. (See chapter 6.) The authors of this study surmised that part of the action of this formula may be via inhibition of arachidonic acid metabolites.[36]

Vitamin E. Vitamin E is a powerful antioxidant that protects cell membranes against excessive damage from free radicals. It is also an essential factor in preventing blood essential fatty acids from undergoing oxidation. Vitamin E is able to block the enzymes phospholipase A2, lipoxygenase, and cyclo-oxygenase, thereby preventing the release of inflammatory prostaglandins.[37,38]

Selenium. Selenium is an important part of the anti-oxidant defense system because it is a critical element in the enzyme glutathione peroxidase. This enzyme protects the body's essential fatty acids from destruction. Selenium has a complementary relationship with vitamin E. It potentiates the effects of vitamin E and may compensate to an extent for deficiency of vitamin E.

Zinc. Zinc has many roles to play in the body. It is needed for proper function of delta-6-desaturase and the conversion of fatty acids into prostaglandins. Zinc is also an inhibitor of lipoxygenase and therefore prevents the formation of leukotrienes.[39] The role of zinc deficiency in recurrent otitis media has been described in chapter 5.

GLA (gamma Linolenic acid). GLA is a known inhibitor of the inflammatory response. It blocks inflammation by undergoing conversion into the anti-inflammatory PGE1. GLA supplementation may be especially important in children with a history of allergy or eczema. Any child who presents with signs of fatty acid deficiency who also has evidence of delta-6-desaturase inhibition (based on a history of exposure to d-6-d inhibitors) may require supplementation with GLA in addition to linoleic acid. The effective dose in children has been shown to be one capsule per day per year of age up to a maximum of six capsules. Some children who do not respond at this dose may require substantially more.[40]

EPA (eicosapentaenoic acid). EPA is incorporated into the membranes of cells, where it displaces arachidonic acid.This reduces the amount of arachidonic acid (or substrate) available for the inflammatory response. EPA is converted into PGE3, exerting an inhibitory effect on the enzymes cyclo-oxygenase and lipoxygenase. EPA also appears to potentiate the effect of the other anti-inflammatory prostaglandin, PGE1.[41] Any child who presents with signs of fatty acid deficiency who also has evidence of delta-6-desaturase inhibition (based on a history of exposure to d-6-d inhibitors) may require supplementation with EPA in addition to linolenic acid.

Beta-Carotene. Beta-carotene, also known as pro-vitamin A, has at least two important functions. Beta-carotene itself is an important anti-oxidant. Clearly, the anti-oxidants do not work alone, but in concert with one another. Therefore, it is important that all anti-oxidants be present in adequate amounts. Beta-carotene is also important because a percentage of dietary beta-carotene undergoes conversion to vitamin A. The importance of vitamin A in otitis media has already been discussed. Both vitamin A and beta-carotene should be present in the diet since the conversion of beta-carotene to vitamin A is believed by some to be insufficient to supply all the vitamin A needs.

A Consideration: Fetal Alcohol Syndrome
In chapter 5, I described the many factors that, individually or in concert, interfere with the proper conversion of fatty acids by blocking the enzyme delta-6-desaturase, Dr. David Horrobin has shown that infants have a poorly developed d-6-d system. He has also shown that intake of alcohol causes the enzyme to be blocked. Since roughly 10 percent of all calories consumed by people in North America are in the form of alcohol,[42] an important question is raised

regarding Fetal Alcohol Syndrome (FAS).

FAS is a condition that affects children born to mothers who have consumed alcohol during the gestational period. The understanding of this syndrome today relates primarily to behavior and motor problems, and to growth irregularities. FAS was originally believed to affect children of alcoholic mothers. However, we now know that even moderate alcohol consumption during pregnancy (as few as one or two drinks) can lead to varying degrees of FAS.

Here is the connection. Alcohol adversely affects the enzyme delta-6-desaturase and can produce significant adverse changes in the children of mothers who consume alcohol just before conception or during pregnancy. Given this, it is conceivable that one of the manifestations of FAS might be impaired fatty acid metabolism due to poorly functioning enzymes. Impaired fatty acid metabolism would, in part, explain some of the behavioral and motor problems of FAS children, since the nervous system is highly dependent upon the proper metabolism of fats. (Obviously, there are numerous additional factors that go beyond this.)

FAS is now as prevalent as Down syndrome (between one in 500 and one in 1,000 births).[43, 44] Children with FAS have an incidence of otitis media equivalent to children with Down syndrome and cleft palate.[45] In addition, there may be a substantial population of children who do not have classic signs of FAS, yet have been adversely affected by mild or moderate consumption of alcohol by the mother. These children would not be recognized as having FAS. Yet there may be sufficient enzyme impairment to significantly disrupt their normal fatty acid metabolism. This would result in a condition favoring inflammation. Theoretically, these children would be at greater risk to inflammatory conditions such as otitis media.

Children with defective d-6-d enzymes would not be expected to respond to any conventional therapy (such as antibiotics or surgery) because they would suffer from an inherent inability to combat inflammation. In such children, even supplementation with linoleic acid, linolenic acid, and co-factors would fail because the enzymes would be unable to convert the fatty acids into PGE1, PGE3, and related compounds. Most likely, substantial amounts

GLA, EPA, and co-factors would be required. This would by-pass the step where d-6-d is required and provide the needed raw material to manufacture PG1 and PG3.* (See figure 19.) Presently this idea is only a hypothesis. It, however, deserves consideration since up to 93 percent of children with FAS suffer from recurrent otitis media.[46]

Nutrition and Immune Function

Nutrition is rapidly being shown to play a crucial role in many aspects of immune function. There are solid indications that nutritional supplementation can have a direct and significant effect on the outcome of infection. Below is a discussion of nutrients known to play a role in immune function.

Zinc. Zinc is perhaps the most extensively researched nutrient with regard to immune function. Deficiency adversely affects T and B-cell function, thymic size and resistance to viruses, bacteria, and parasites. Zinc deficiency can impair both the primary and secondary immune response.[47,48,49,50,51,52] It has been estimated that roughly three-fourths of the American population are zinc-deficient.[53]

Copper. Copper deficiency has been associated with decreased immune competence and increased incidence of infection.[54] Excessive zinc intake can lead to copper deficiency. Excessive zinc levels sometimes occur in individuals who are taking zinc as a supplement. Copper excess has also been linked to immune impairment. When copper is present in excessive amounts, it exerts an antagonistic effect on zinc, leading to zinc deficiency.

Selenium. Deficiency of selenium results in diminished resistance to microbial and viral infections, neutrophil function, antibody pro-

---

*This additional need for GLA and EPA should also be considered in diabetic children who suffer from recurrent otitis media. Juvenile onset diabetes is complex and should be managed carefully. Any nutritional changes should only be undertaken after consultation with a doctor.

duction, and reduced ability of T-cells and natural killer cells to destroy pathogens. Supplementation with selenium has been shown to reverse these processes. This trace element has been said to "... affect all components of the immune system."[55]

This additional need for GLA and EPA should also be considered in diabetic children who suffer from recurrent otitis media. Juvenile onset diabetes is complex and should be managed carefully. Any nutritional changes should only be undertaken after consultation with a doctor.

Germanium. Germanium is an immune-potentiating trace element when used therapeutically. Germanium is known to stimulate interferon production and is considered an immune-regulator. It is believed to have anti-oxidant properties as well.[56]

Vitamin C. The effects of vitamin C on immune function have been widely publicized. Vitamin C appears to stimulate interferon production, enhance T-lymphocyte function, enhance antibody formation, and reduce the adverse effects of environmental chemicals. Vitamin C plays an important role in white cell phagocytosis.[57] Esterified L-ascorbic acid appears to be the most effective for use in acute infections when rapid uptake is required. Recent evidence suggests that ingestion of esterified ascorbic acid results in twice the blood levels and four times the tissue levels when compared to ascorbate and citrate forms. Esterified forms are also excreted less rapidly, which is desirable when lasting action is needed.[58]

Bioflavonoids. The bioflavonoid quercitin has been shown to inhibit the replication of several viruses including herpes simplex type 1, polio virus type 1, parainfluenzal virus type 3, and respiratory syncytial virus.[59, 60]

Vitamin E. Vitamin E exerts an effect on the immune system through its role as an antioxidant. It also affects immune function by regulating the formation of prostaglandins. Vitamin E exerts a protective effect on vitamin A. Also, when vitamin E is deficient, vitamin

A absorption is impaired.[61, 62] Excessive vitamin E intake has an immunosuppressive effect,though this is controversial.[63]

Pyridoxine. Pyridoxine deficiency results in depressed humoral and cell-mediated immunity and inhibition of the antibody response.[64] Anecdotal reports have shown an increased incidence of otitis media associated with pyridoxine deficiency. Supplementation of pyridoxine should not be undertaken without adequate B-vitamins, since conversion of pyridoxine to the active pyridoxal-5-phosphate requires riboflavin and may require other nutrients.

Beta-carotene. Beta-carotene is one of the most potent free-radical scavengers yet discovered. It is of major importance in protecting the cellular lining of the lungs and respiratory tract. There is evidence that it plays a similar role in the lining of the eustachian tube and tympanic cavity. Modest doses appear to stimulate the immune response.[65]

Vitamin A. Vitamin A deficiency results in thymic and splenic atrophy, and a reduction in the numbers of circulating leukocytes and lymphocytes.[66] Supplementation may reverse these effects. Excessive vitamin A (retinol or retinoic acid) can be immunosuppressive.[67] Whenever vitamin A is given therapeutically, beta-carotene should also be given. Beta-carotene appears to prevent the macrophage inhibition that can occur with vitamin A supplementation.

Fat. Excessive fat intake or elevated blood fats (cholesterol or triglycerides) tend to decrease resistance to bacterial and viral infections.[68] Linoleic acid, linolenic acid, and eicosapentaenoic acid all have been shown to have anti-bacterial, anti-fungal, and anti-viral activity.[69]

Pantothenic acid. Pantothenic acid is a water-soluble vitamin that is greatly affected by stress and illness. During these times, the adrenal glands require large amounts of pantothenic acid. When pantothenic acid is deficient, the adrenal glands begin to atrophy.[70]

During deficiency there is an increased susceptibility to infection, decrease in gamma globulin concentrations, impaired antigenic response, and poor viral and bacterial defenses.[71, 72]

Thymus tissue. Within the past ten years, substantial documentation has confirmed the value of raw bovine thymus tissue supplementation in cases of recurrent infections and decreased immunocompetence. Ingestion of oral thymus tissue can enhance T and B lymphocyte formation, increase T helper levels and activity, and balance T helper/suppressor ratios.[73,74,75] Bovine thymus tissue is known to contain thymosin, serum thymic factor, thymopoieten, and other biologically active substances.[76] Thymus tissue appears to be effective in the treatment of acute and chronic infections. Only thymus tissue that has been defatted or azeotrophically processed should be used because of the possibility of contamination by bovine slow viruses.[77]

* * *

There is yet no standard or accepted protocol for the nutritional management of otitis media. This is because our understanding of nutrition as it relates to inflammation/infection is only now emerging. The second reason is that the possibility of a nutritional role in otitis media has gained little attention within the medical community. While deficiency of certain nutrients seem to be common in recurrent otitis media, there are a host of other nutritional factors that may be important in a given child. Therefore, this final chapter is intended as a starting point.

The nutritional recommendations given in chapter 6 are based on a general knowledge of nutrition and immunity, and nutrition and inflammation. It is a basic approach that may be helpful for some children. The practitioner who is confronted with a child with recurrent otitis media must consider the full range of diagnostic possibilities—both nutritional and otherwise. Any therapeutic nutritional program that is undertaken should be done concurrently with an elimination of anti-nutrients such as trans fatty acids, heavy metals, sugar, and others.

Epilogue

Middle ear problems consume enormous time, energy, and resources from both parents and the medical system. It is clear from the evidence that we must take a radical turn in our approach to treating this disorder.

If it is true that the majority of children with earaches improve on their own, then we should let this benign illness run its course where appropriate. If there are repeated cases that do not resolve, we should investigate every avenue of conservative care before resorting to costly or invasive procedures with unproven benefit.

European countries are far more reluctant to rush to aggressive drug and surgical intervention. This approach has benefited their children and their medical system greatly. Perhaps we should follow their lead and end the unjustifiable reliance on antibiotic drugs. For if we do not, nature will surely end it for us, as evidenced by the disturbing increase in drug-resistant bacteria.

In choosing treatment for this disorder, we should look to more fundamental mechanisms. We should determine the factors that have rendered a child susceptible to invasion by bacteria (or viruses). We should consider that the interaction between humans and the microbial world is complex and that integrated treatments are often required. We should understand that diet, nutrition, lifestyle, genetic, environment, and psychological factors all interact to tip the scales in favor of child or microbe.

Our knowledge of diet and nutrition is growing at a breathtaking rate. While the number of physicians who've taken notice has grown, few have integrated the advances into their daily practice.

As the level of sophistication of this nutrition knowledge increases, our ability to ask complex questions and devise targeted treatment increases. Yet, even as our nutrition knowledge grows the quality of the childhood diet seems in decline. Thus, the call to intervention in this area becomes more urgent.

As we grapple with rapid environmental changes, novel chemical compounds, and an increasingly polluted environment, we must recognize the unique susceptibility of children. We must also recognize that when the nutritional status of children is compromised their ability to remain protected in the face of environmental insult declines.

As we grapple with the growing stresses of childhood in the modern age, we must remain aware of the voluminous evidence showing the effect of psychological factors on immune defense and susceptibility to infection.

Natural medicine has, for many decades (indeed centuries), managed childhood illness with grace and elegance. Childhood ear infection has shown itself to be responsive to many of the modalities of what we now call complementary or natural medicine. We should be willing to entertain the notion that sophisticated natural healing systems have evolved over time to provide some solutions to complex medical problems. When we open our minds to move beyond the limits of our own training, we are able to see that there are many paths to health and wellbeing. We are able to see that no one system holds the answer for all people at all times. Realizing this allows us to truly see the valuable in all healing systems and to use that which best suits an individual.

The modern child is faced with more opportunity than perhaps ever before. Yet the challenges are great. We cannot afford to allow illness early in life to cloud a child's future. The cost to the individual, to families, and to society are significant. Yet, reliance on aggressive medical therapy for children with uncomplicated illness may do just that.

To stem the rising tide of ear infections in children, we must enlist the help of all people, including parents, doctors, day care providers, educators, and public health officials. As a society, we must redefine our lifestyles and change our eating habits. Parents must demand that their doctors be knowledgeable in the intricacies of nutritional medicine and open to methods that have a rich cultural history of benefit.

I believe it is time to look beyond the microbe. There is no doubt that bacteria and viruses exact a considerable toll on human health. We must be ever aware of their capacity to wreak havoc and cause illness. But for far too long, doctors have ignored the important role of the host. Medical officials suggest that we are moving into the "post-antibiotic era where untreatable infections will again be seen." Yet, no one has yet described the future of this new world.

While all journeys contain uncertainty, mystery, and, perhaps, danger, I propose that we chart our own course. I propose that we move into the era of **host defenses.** In this new era, we will utilize our sophisticated knowledge to bolster immune defenses and summon the considerable abilities of the human body to heal itself. This is one of the next great frontiers. It promises to be a journey of excitement and drama.

Appendix

Resources

Listed below are companies that sell various health-related products. This list is not an endorsement of any company or product. It is for informational purposes only. Note that some companies market only to health care professionals and prefer not to respond to inquiries from the public. These are indicated with an asterisk.

Nutritional Products

Nutrition Dynamics
Consumer Division
5410 Highway 12
Maple Plain, MN 55359
800-444-9998

Nutrition Dynamics has a wide range of nutritional products by different manufacturers. They are a reputable company that does business with the public.

Ethical Nutrients
971 Calle Negocio
San Clemente, CA 92873

NutriCology, Inc.
400 Preda Street
San Leandro, CA ¨94577
800-545-9960

Spectrum Naturals
133 Copeland Street
Petaluma, CA 94952
707-778-8900

Homeopathic Medicine

Biological Homeopathic
Industries*
11600 Cochiti S.E.
Albuquerque, NM 87123
800-621-7644

Boiron-Bornemann
1208 Amosland Road
Norwood, PA 19074
800-258-8823

Homeopathic Educational
  Services
2124 Kittredge Avenue
Berkeley, CA 94704
510-649-0294 (inquiries)
800-359-9051 (orders)

Boericke & Tafel, Inc.
2381 Circadian Way
Santa Rosa, CA 95407
800-876-9505

Standard Homeopathic Co.
210 W.131st Street
Los Angeles, CA 90061
800-624-9659

Botanical Medicine

K'an Herb ¨Company*
2425 Porter Street, Suite 18
Soquel, CA ¨95073
800-543-5233

Brion Herb Corporation*
12020 B.Centralia Rd.
Hawaiian Gardens, CA 90716
800-333-HERB

I.T.M.*
2442 S.E.Sherman
Portland, OR 97214
800-544-7504

McZand Herbal, Inc.*
P.O.Box 5312
Santa Monica, CA 90405
213-392-8404

Acupuncture

OMS Medical Supplies, Inc.*
1950 Washington Street
Braintree, MA 02184
800-323-1839

Redwing Book Company
44 Linden Street
Brookline, MA 02146
800-873-3946

Organizations

American Academy of
  Environmental Medicine
P.O. Box 16106
Denver, CO 80216

Candida Research Information
  Foundation
P.O. Box 2719
Castro Valley, CA 94546
(415) 582–2179

Human Ecology Action League
  (HEAL)
P.O. Box 66637
Chicago, IL 60666
(312) 665–6575

International Health Foundation
William Crook, M.D.
800–372-7665

American Holistic Medical
  Association
2727 Fairview Avenue E.
Seattle, WA 98102
(206) 322–6842

International College of
  Applied Kinesiology
10540 Marty, Suite 240
Shawnee Mission, KS 66212
(913) 648–2828

American Chiropractic
  Association
1701 Clarendon Boulevard.
Arlington, VA 22209

American Osteopathic
  Association
212 East Ohio Street
Chicago, IL 60611
(312) 280–5800

National Resources Defense
  Council
800–648-NRDC

National Center for
  Homeopathy
1500 Massachusetts Avenue N.W.
Washington, DC 20005
(202) 223–6182

American Institute of
  Homeopathy
1500 Massachusetts Avenue N.W.
Washington, DC 20005

International Foundation for
  Homeopathy
2366 Eastlake Avenue E. #301
Seattle, WA 98102

British Homeopathic
Association
27A Devonshire Street
London, W1N 1RJ, England

Foundation for Homeopathic
    Education & Research
5916 Chabot Crest
Oakland, CA 94618
(415) 649–8930

National Commission for the
    Certification of
    Acupuncturists
1424 16th Street N.W.
Suite 501
Washington, DC 20036
(202) 323–1404

American Academy of
    Acupuncture and Oriental
    Medicine
1424 16th Street N.W.
Suite 501
Washington, DC 20036
(202) 265–2287

Institute for Traditional
Medicine
2017 S.E. Hawthorne
Portland, OR 97214
800–544-7504

Nutrition Assessment Using Laboratory

The nutritional status of any child can be measured using a variety of means. Development of new laboratory tests has allowed doctors to evalutate the complex interaction among vitamins, minerals, fatty acids, amino acids, and intermediate compounds.

This appendix contains the laboratory report of a three-year-old named Sarah who has Down syndrome and repeated infections. You will notice that many substances are out of the reference range, either high or low. You would expect a child with this degree of biochemical abnormality to have physical and psychological problems. Other children with Down syndrome show similarities with regard to some lab values while other values are unique to the individual.

Using tests such as this, doctors have been able to tailor nutritional therapies best suited to the individual child. In Sarah's case, nutritional therapy has resulted in significant and consistent improvement in her health status. Similar tests can be used to assess the health status of any child.

MetaMetrix Medical Laboratory
5000 Peachtree Ind. Blvd., Suite 110, Norcross, GA 30071
(404) 446-5483 • Fax (404) 441-2237

Accession Number	41434
Report Status	FINAL
Report Page	1

Physician Name and Address

Patient Name

Age	Sex	Clinical Information
3	F	

Date Specimen Collected	Date Specimen Received	Report Date
4/13/95	4/14/95	4/24/95

Physician Telephone	Physician Fax Number	Tech. No.
		P 0

Comments

T22

TEST	RESULTS		LIMITS

Minerals Analysis - Erythrocyte

Method: Inductively Coupled Plasma Emission Spectroscopy and Stable Temperature Platform Furnace Atomic Absorption Spectros copy

Copper	0.75	µg/ml erythrocytes	0.5 - 1.8
Potassium	2982		2500 - 4500
Magnesium	54		40 - 65
Zinc	13.1		6 - 20
Manganese	0.02	L	0.05 - 0.25
Selenium	0.26		0.18 - 0.7

Serum Lipid Peroxides

Method: High Pressure Liquid Chromatography

Serum Lipid Peroxides	1.7	mg/dL	H	≤ 1.25

Vitamins A, E, & Carotene

Method: High Pressure Liquid Chromatography

Vitamin A	64	µg/dL		40 - 95
Vitamin E	5.9	mg/L	L	10 - 25
β Carotene	9	µg/dL	L	20 - 85

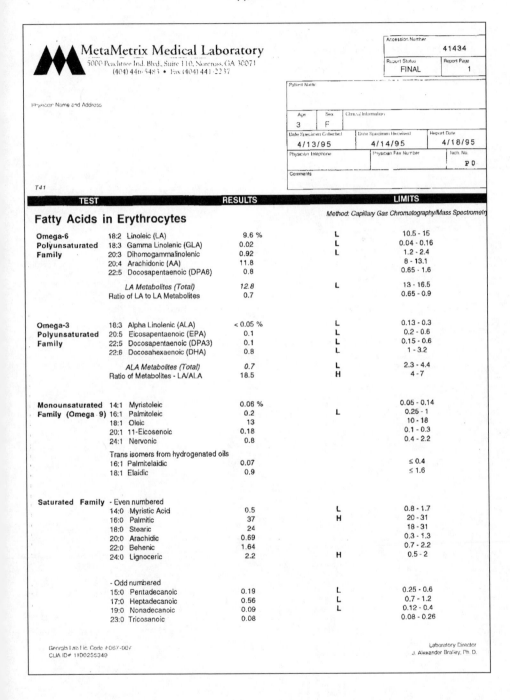

MetaMetrix Medical Laboratory
5000 Peachtree Ind. Blvd., Suite 110, Norcross, GA 30071
(404) 446-5483 • Fax (404) 441-2237

Accession Number	41434
Report Status	FINAL
Report Page	1

Physician Name and Address

Patient Name:

Age	Sex	Clinical Information
3	F	

Date Specimen Collected	Date Specimen Received	Report Date
4/13/95	4/14/95	4/18/95

Physician Telephone	Physician Fax Number	Tech. No.
		P 0

Comments

T41

TEST	RESULTS	LIMITS

Fatty Acids in Erythrocytes

Method: Capillary Gas Chromatography/Mass Spectrometry

Omega-6 Polyunsaturated Family

18:2	Linoleic (LA)	9.6 %	L	10.5 - 15
18:3	Gamma Linolenic (GLA)	0.02	L	0.04 - 0.16
20:3	Dihomogammalinolenic	0.92	L	1.2 - 2.4
20:4	Arachidonic (AA)	11.8		8 - 13.1
22:5	Docosapentaenoic (DPA6)	0.8		0.65 - 1.6
	LA Metabolites (Total)	*12.8*	L	13 - 16.5
	Ratio of LA to LA Metabolites	0.7		0.65 - 0.9

Omega-3 Polyunsaturated Family

18:3	Alpha Linolenic (ALA)	< 0.05 %	L	0.13 - 0.3
20:5	Eicosapentaenoic (EPA)	0.1	L	0.2 - 0.6
22:5	Docosapentaenoic (DPA3)	0.1	L	0.15 - 0.6
22:6	Docosahexaenoic (DHA)	0.8	L	1 - 3.2
	ALA Metabolites (Total)	*0.7*	L	2.3 - 4.4
	Ratio of Metabolites - LA/ALA	18.5	H	4 - 7

Monounsaturated Family (Omega 9)

14:1	Myristoleic	0.06 %		0.05 - 0.14
16:1	Palmitoleic	0.2	L	0.25 - 1
18:1	Oleic	13		10 - 18
20:1	11-Eicosenoic	0.18		0.1 - 0.3
24:1	Nervonic	0.8		0.4 - 2.2

Trans isomers from hydrogenated oils

16:1	Palmitelaidic	0.07		≤ 0.4
18:1	Elaidic	0.9		≤ 1.6

Saturated Family - Even numbered

14:0	Myristic Acid	0.5	L	0.8 - 1.7
16:0	Palmitic	37	H	20 - 31
18:0	Stearic	24		18 - 31
20:0	Arachidic	0.69		0.3 - 1.3
22:0	Behenic	1.64		0.7 - 2.2
24:0	Lignoceric	2.2	H	0.5 - 2

- Odd numbered

15:0	Pentadecanoic	0.19	L	0.25 - 0.6
17:0	Heptadecanoic	0.56	L	0.7 - 1.2
19:0	Nonadecanoic	0.09	L	0.12 - 0.4
23:0	Tricosanoic	0.08		0.08 - 0.26

Georgia Lab Lic. Code #067-007
CLIA ID# 11D0255349

Laboratory Director
J. Alexander Bralley, Ph. D.

MetaMetrix Medical Laboratory
5000 Peachtree Ind. Blvd., Suite 110, Norcross, GA 30071
(404) 446-5483 • Fax (404) 441-2237

Physician Name and Address

Accession Number	41434
Report Status	FINAL
Report Page	1

Patient Name		
Age	Sex	Clinical Information
3	F	

Date Specimen Collected	Date Specimen Received	Report Date
4/13/95	4/14/95	5/19/95

Physician Telephone	Physician Fax Number	Test No.
		P 0

Comments

T11

TEST	RESULTS	LIMITS

Amino Acid Analysis - 20 Plasma

Method: High Pressure Liquid Chromatography

		RESULTS		LIMITS
ESSENTIAL AMINO ACIDS	Arginine	340 µmol/L		200 - 700
	Histidine	41	L	50 - 140
	Isoleucine	62		40 - 120
	Leucine	28	L	125 - 280
	Lysine	86		70 - 150
	Methionine	35		25 - 50
	Phenylalanine	50	L	55 - 140
	Threonine	74		65 - 250
	Tryptophan	57		50 - 120
	Valine	203		160 - 420
ESSENTIAL AMINO ACID DERIVATIVES				
Neuroendocrine Metabolism	Glycine	256		180 - 450
	Serine	91		90 - 200
	Taurine	47		45 - 250
	Tyrosine	29	L	30 - 120
Ammonia/Energy Metabolism	Asparagine	5	L	40 - 100
	Aspartic acid	17		5 - 30
	Citrulline	20	L	25 - 60
	Glutamic acid	45		30 - 150
	Glutamine	141	L	350 - 950
	Ornithine	15	L	30 - 90

Georgia Lab Lic. Code #067-007
CLIA ID# 11D0255349

Laboratory Director
J. Alexander Bralley, Ph. D.

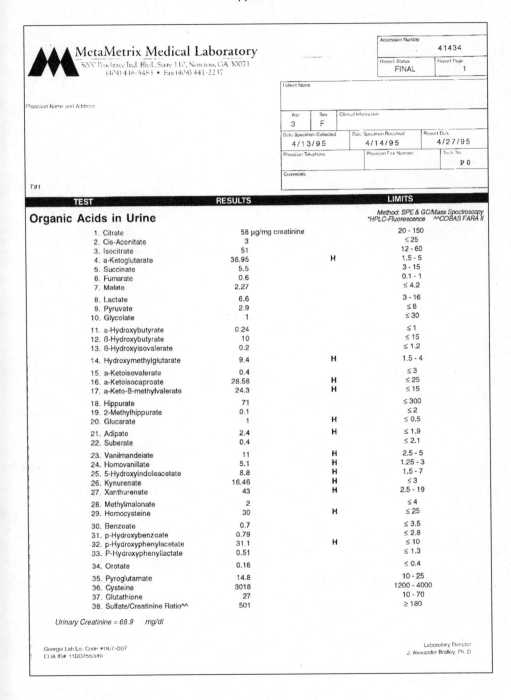

MetaMetrix Medical Laboratory
5000 Peachtree Ind. Blvd., Suite 110, Norcross, GA 30071
(404) 446-5483 • Fax (404) 441-2237

Physician Name and Address

T91

Accession Number		41434
Report Status FINAL		Report Page 1

Patient Name			
Age 3	Sex F	Clinical Information	
Date Specimen Collected 4/13/95	Date Specimen Received 4/14/95		Report Date 4/27/95
Physician Telephone	Physician Fax Number		Tech No P 0
Comments			

TEST	RESULTS		LIMITS

Organic Acids in Urine

Method: SPE & GC/Mass Spectroscopy
*HPLC-Fluorescence   ^^COBAS FARA II

1. Citrate	58 µg/mg creatinine		20 - 150
2. Cis-Aconitate	3		≤ 25
3. Isocitrate	51		12 - 60
4. a-Ketoglutarate	38.95	H	1.5 - 5
5. Succinate	5.5		3 - 15
6. Fumarate	0.6		0.1 - 1
7. Malate	2.27		≤ 4.2
8. Lactate	6.6		3 - 16
9. Pyruvate	2.9		≤ 8
10. Glycolate	1		≤ 30
11. a-Hydroxybutyrate	0.24		≤ 1
12. ß-Hydroxybutyrate	10		≤ 15
13. ß-Hydroxyisovalerate	0.2		≤ 1.2
14. Hydroxymethylglutarate	9.4	H	1.5 - 4
15. a-Ketoisovalerate	0.4		≤ 3
16. a-Ketoisocaproate	28.58	H	≤ 25
17. a-Keto-ß-methylvalerate	24.3	H	≤ 15
18. Hippurate	71		≤ 300
19. 2-Methylhippurate	0.1		≤ 2
20. Glucarate	1	H	≤ 0.5
21. Adipate	2.4	H	≤ 1.9
22. Suberate	0.4		≤ 2.1
23. Vanilmandelate	11	H	2.5 - 5
24. Homovanillate	5.1	H	1.25 - 3
25. 5-Hydroxyindoleacetate	8.8	H	1.5 - 7
26. Kynurenate	16.46	H	≤ 3
27. Xanthurenate	43	H	2.5 - 19
28. Methylmalonate	2		≤ 4
29. Homocysteine	30	H	≤ 25
30. Benzoate	0.7		≤ 3.5
31. p-Hydroxybenzoate	0.79		≤ 2.8
32. p-Hydroxyphenylacetate	31.1	H	≤ 10
33. P-Hydroxyphenyllactate	0.51		≤ 1.3
34. Orotate	0.16		≤ 0.4
35. Pyroglutamate	14.8		10 - 25
36. Cysteine	3018		1200 - 4000
37. Glutathione	27		10 - 70
38. Sulfate/Creatinine Ratio^^	501		≥ 180

Urinary Creatinine = 68.9   mg/dl

Georgia Lab Lic. Code #067-007
CLIA ID# 11D0255349

Laboratory Director
J. Alexander Bralley, Ph. D

References

Introduction

1. Diamant, M.; Diamant, B.; "Abuse and Timing of Use of Antibiotics in Acute Otitis Media," *Arch. Otolaryngol.* 100:226–232, 1974.

2. Van Buchem, F.L.; "Therapy of Acute Otitis Media: Myringotomy, Antibiotics, or Neither? A Double-Blind Study in Children," *Lancet* 883, Oct. 24, 1981.

3. Chaput de Saintonge, D.M.; Levine, D.F.; et al.; "Trial of Three-Day and Ten-Day Courses of Amoxycillin in Otitis Media," *Br. Med. J.* 284, Apr. 10, 1982.

4. Brown, M.J.; Richards, S.H.; Ambegaoker, A.G.; "Grommets and Glue Ear: A Five-Year Follow-Up of a Controlled Trial," *J. Roy. Soc. Med.* 71:353–356, 1978.

5. Pang, L.Q.; "The Importance of Allergy in Otolaryngology," *Clinical Ecology*, Dickey, L. (Ed.), Charles Thomas, Springfield, Illinois, p. 633, 1976.

6. Skoner, D.P.; Stillwagon, P.K.; et al.; "Inflammatory Mediators in Chronic Otitis Media with Effusion," *Arch. Otolaryngol. Head Neck Surg.* 114:1131–1133, Oct., 1988.

7. Bondestam, M.; Foucard, T.; Gebre-Medhin, M.; "Subclinical Trace Element Deficiency in Children with Undue Susceptibility to Infections," *Act. Paed. Sc.* 74:515–520, 1985.

Chapter 1. The Scope of the Problem

1. Eisenberg, L.; "Preventive Pediatrics: The Promise and the Peril," *Pediatrics* 80 (3): pp. 415–416, 1987.

2. Asman, B.J.; Fireman, P.; "The Role of Allergies in the Development of Otitis Media with Effusion," *Intl. Ped.* 3 (3):231–233, July-Sept., 1988.

3. Teele, D.W.; Klein, J.O.; Rosner, B.A.; "Epidemiology of Otitis Media in Children," *Ann-Otol-Rhinol-Laryngol* [Suppl.] 89 (3 Pt 2 Suppl. 68):5–6, May-June, 1980.

4. American Academy of Otolaryngology Head and Neck Surgery, 1101 Vermont Ave. N.W., Suite 302, Washington, D.C. 20005, 1989.

5. Cantekin, E. The case against aggressive, expensive, and ineffective treatment of a benign disease: Comments on the clinical practice

guidelines on otitis media. Report submitted to the U.S. Congress and the Department of Health and Human Services. 1, 1994.

6. Teele, D.W.; Klein, J.O.; Rosner, B.A.; "Epidemiology of Otitis Media in Children," *Ann-Otol-Rhinol-Laryngol* [Suppl.] 89(3 Pt 2 Suppl. 68):5–6, 1980.

7. Eichenwald, H.E.; "Otitis Media in the Child," *Hospital Practice* May 30, 1985.

8. Froom, J.; "Otitis Media: Clinical Review," *J. Fam. Pract.* 15(4): 1982.

9. Schappert, S.: Office visits for otitis media in the United States, 1975–1990. Advance Data 214:1–15, 1992.

10. Paparella, M.M.; "Complications and Sequelae of Otitis Media: State of the Art," in Lim DJ (ed.) *Recent Advances in Otitis Media with Effusion*. Burlington, Ontario, Canada, BC Decker, Inc., pp. 316–319, 1984.

11. Halsted, C.; Lepow, M.L.; Bosassamian, N.; "Otitis Media: Clinical Observations, Microbiology and Evaluation of Therapy," *Am. J. Dis. Child.* 115:542, 1968.

12. Biles, R.W.; Buffler, P.A.; O'Donell, A.A.; "Epidemiology of Otitis Media: A Community Study," *Am. J. Pub. Hlth.* 70:593, 1980.

13. Saarinen, U.; "Breastfeeding Prevents Otitis Media," *Nutrition Reviews* 41(8):241, Aug., 1983.

14. Teele, D.W.; Klein, J.O.; Rosner, B.A.; "Epidemiology of Otitis Media in Children," *Ann-Otol-Rhinol-Laryngol* [Suppl]. May-June, 89 (3 Pt 2 Suppl. 68), pp. 5–6, 1980.

15. Kraemer, M.J.; Richardson, M.A.; et al.; "Risk Factors for Persistent Middle Ear Effusions: Otitis Media, Catarrh, Cigarette Smoke Exposure and Atopy," *J.A.M.A.* 249(8):1022–5, Feb. 25, 1983.

16. Church, M.W.; Gerkin, K.P.; "Hearing Disorders in Children with Fetal Alcohol Syndrome: Findings From Case Reports," *Pediatrics* 82(2):147–154, 1988.

17. Schwartz, D.M.; Schwartz, R.H.; "Acoustic Impedance and Otoscopic Findings in Young Children with Down's Syndrome," *Arch. Otoloaryngol.* 104:652, 1978.

18. Backman, A.; Bjorksten, F.; et al.; "Do Infections in Infancy Affect Sensitization to Airborne Allergens and Development of Atopic Disease? A Retrospective Study of Seven-Year-Old Children," *Allergy* 39(4):309–15, May, 1984.

19. Draper, W.L.; "Secretory Otitis Media," *Clinical Ecology*, Dickey, L. (Ed.), Charles Thomas, Springfield, Illinois, pp. 176–178, 1976.

20. Bondestam, M.; Foucard, T.; Gebre-Medhin, M.; "Subclinical Trace

Element Deficiency in Children with Undue Susceptibility to Infections," *Act. Paed. Sc.* 74:515–520, 1985.

21. "Report of a Survey by the Medical Research Council's Working-party for Research in General Practice: Acute Otitis Media in General Practice," *Lancet* 2:510, 1957.

22. Gutmann, G.; "Das Atlas-Blockierungs-Syndrome des Sauglings und des Kleinkindes," *Manuelle Med.* 25:5–10, 1987.

23. Howie, V.M.; Ploussard, J.H.; Sloyer, J.; "The 'Otitis-Prone' Condition," *Am. J. Dis. Child.* 129:676–8, 1975.

24. Roberts, J.E.; Burchinal, M.R.; et al.; "Otitis Media in Early Childhood and Cognitive, Academic, and Classroom Performance of the School-Aged Child," *Pediatrics* 83(4): 1989.

25. Paradise, J.L.; "Management of Secretory Otitis Media: State of the Art," *Adv. Oto-Rhino-Laryng.* 40:103, 1988.

26. Stool, S.; et al.: "Otitis Media with Effusion." U.S. Department of Health and Human Services, AHCPR Publication No. 94-0622, 1994.

27. Ibid.

28. Jung, T.T.K.; "Arachidonic Acid Metabolites in Otitis Media Pathogenesis," *Ann. Otol. Rhinol. Laryngol.* 97:1988.

29. Doran, T.F.; DeAngelis, C.; Baumgardner, R.A.; Mellitis, E.D.; "Acetaminophen: More Harm Than Good for Chickenpox?" *J. Pediatrics* 114(6):1045–8, 1989.

30. Stool, S.; et al.: "Otitis Media with Effusion." U.S. Department of Health and Human Services, AHCPR Publication No. 94-0622, 53, 1994.

31. Ibid.

32. Ibid.

33. Sade, J.; *Secretory Otitis Media and Its Sequelae.* Churchill Livingstone, Inc., 1979.

34. Fiellau-Nikolajsen, M.; "Adenoidectomy for Eustachian Tube Dysfunction: Long-term Results from a Randomized Controlled Trial," *Acta. Otolaryngol.* Suppl., 386:129, 1982.

35. Widemar, L.; "The Effect of Adenoidectomy on Secretory Otitis Media," *Acta. Otolaryngol.* Suppl., 386:132, 1983.

36. Stool, S.; et al.: "Otitis Media with Effusion." U.S. Department of Health and Human Services, AHCPR Publication No. 94–0622, 1994.

37. Sadé, J.; Luntz, M.: "Adenoidectomy in Otitis Media: A Review." *Ann. Otol. Rhinol. Laryngol.* 100:226–31, 1991.

38. Bluestone, C.D.; et al.; "Controversies in Antimicrobial Agents for Otitis Media," *Ann. Otol. Rhinol. Laryngol.* Suppl., 1988.

39. Cantekin, E.: The case against aggressive, expensive, and ineffective treatment of a benign disease: Comments on the clinical practice guidelines on otitis media. Report submitted to the U.S. Congress and the Department of Health and Human Services. 50, 1994.

40. Paradise, J.L.; "Management of Secretory Otitis Media: State of the Art," *Adv. Oto-Rhino-Laryng.* 40:99–109, 1988.

41. Samuels, M.; Samuels, N.; *The Well Baby Book*, Summit Books, N.Y., pp. 270–272, 1979.

42. Van Buchem, F.L.; Peeters, M.F.; Van't Hof, M.A.: "Acute Otitis Media: A New Treatment Strategy." *Br. Med. J.* 290(6):1033–37, 1985.

43. Shaffer, H.L.; "Acute Masoiditis and Cholesteatoma," *Otolaryngology* 86:394, 1978.

44. Pfaltz, C.R.; "Complications of Acute Otitis Media in Children," *Adv. Oto-Rhino-Laryng.* 40:70–80, 1988.

45. Paparella, M.M.; Goycoolea, M.; et al.; "Silent Otitis Media: Clinical Applications," *Laryngoscope* 96:978–985, Sept. 1986.

46. Froom, J.; "Clinical Review: Otitis Media," *J. Fam. Pract.* 15(4): 743–770, 1982.

47. Consensus inTherapy of acute otitis media, Nederlands Tijdschrift Voor Geneeskunde, 36:85–88, 1992.

48. Glue Ear Guidelines: Time to Act On the Evidence. *Lancet* 340:1324–1325, 1992.

49. Less Surgery for Glue Ear Says Bulletin. *Br. Med.J.* 305:1454–1455, 1992.

50. Consensus Statement, Middle Ear Inflammation in Children, Swedish Planning and Rationalization of Health and Social Services, Swedish Medical Research Council, 1992.

51. Cantekin, E. The case against aggressive, expensive, and ineffective treatment of a benign disease: Comments on the clinical practice guidelines on otitis media. Report submitted to the U.S. Congress and the Department of Health and Human Services. 53–56, 1994.

Chapter 2. Antibiotics: Sensible Use or Abuse?

1. Galland, L.; Buchman, D.D.; *SuperImmunity for Kids*, E.P. Dutton, New York, p. 201, 1988.

2. Lildholdt, T.; "Unilateral Grommet Insertion and Adenoidectomy in Bilateral Secretory Otitis Media: Preliminary Report of the Results in 91 Children," *Clin. Otolaryngol.* 4:87–93, 1979.

3. Fabricious, H.F.; "Hearing Investigation of School Children in North

Trondelay County," *J. Oslo City Hospital* 18:3, 1968.

4. "Pediatric Antibiotic Use Soars (As Adult Prescriptions Slide),"
Medical World News November 9, 1987.

5. Nelson, W.; Conference on Antimicrobial Agents and Chemotherapy, FDA Report, New York, 1987.

6. "Pediatric Antibiotic Use Soars (As Adult Prescriptions Slide),"
Medical World News November 9, 1987.

7. Lappé, M.; *When Antibiotics Fail: Restoring the Ecology of the Body*,
North Atlantic Books, Berkeley, California, 1986.

8. Schwartz, R.; Rodriguez, W.; Khan, W.; Ross, S.; "The Increasing Incidence of Ampicillin-Resistant *Haemophilus influenzae* : A Cause of Otitis Media," *J.A.M.A.* 239(4): Jan. 23, 1978.

9. Georghiou, G.P., "The Magnitude of the Resistance Problem," in NRC, Board of Agriculture, Pesticide Resistance: Strategies and Tactics for Management, National Academy Press, Washington, D.C., 1986.

10. *Drug Information*, American Hospital Formulary Service, American Society of Hospital Pharmacists, Inc., Bethesda, MD, p. 218, 1986.

11. Faden, et al.: *Ann. Otol. Rhinol. Laryngol.* 1992.

12. Welch, H.G.; "Antibiotic Resistance: A New Kind of Epidemic,"
Postgraduate Medicine 76(6): Nov. 1, 1984.

13. Crossley, K.; et al.; "An Outbreak of Infections Caused by Strains of *S. aureus* Resistant to Methicillin and Aminoglycosides," *J. Infect. Dis.* 139:273–87, 1979.

14. Belsheim, J.A.; Gnarpe, G.H.; "Antibiotics and Granulocytes; Direct and Indirect Effects on Granulocyte Chemotaxis," *Acta. Path. Mocrobiol. Scand.* Sect C, 89:217:221, 1981.

15. Nord, C.E.; and Edlund, C.: "Impact of Antimicrobial Agents On Human Intestinal Microflora." *J. Chemotherapy* 2(4):218–37, 1990

16. Gillon, J.; "Protozoan Infections of the GI Tract," *Quart. J. Med.* 52:29–39, 1984.

17. Pickering, L.K.; Woodward, W.E.; "Diarrhea in Day Care Centers," *Ped. Infect. Dis. J.* 1(1):47–51, 1982.

18. Nussenzweigh, R.S.; "Parasitic Disease as a Cause of Immunosuppression," *New Engl. J. Med.* Feb. 18, 1982.

19. Burdon, D.W.; "Treatment of Pseudomembranous Colitis and Antibotic-Associated Diarrhea," *J. Antimicr. Chemoth.* 14 Suppl. D, pp. 103–109, 1984.

20. Helstrom, P.B.; Balish, E.; "Effect of Oral Tetracycline, the Microbial Flora, and the Athymic State on Gastrointestinal Colonization and

Infection of BA1B/c mice with Candida albicans," *Infection and Immunity* pp. 764–74, Mar., 1979.

21. Galland, L.; *SuperImmunity for Kids*, E.P. Dutton, New York, p. 215, 1988.

22. Flores, E.C.; Plumb, S.C.; McNeese, M.C.; "Intestinal Parasitosis in an Urban Pediatric Clinic Population," *Am. J. Dis. Child.* 137: 754–756, 1983.

23. Andre, C.; et al.: "Effect of Allergen Ingestion Challenge With and Without Cromoglycate Cover on Intestinal Permeability in Atopic Dermatitis, Urticaria, and Other Symptoms of Food Allergy." *Allergy* 44(9):47–51, 1989

24. Andre, C.; et al.: "Measurement of intestinal permeability to Mannitol and Lactulose as a Means of Diagnosing Food Allergy and Evaluating Therapeutic Effectiveness of Disodium Cromoglycate." *Annals allergy* 59(II):127–130, 1987.

25. Franco, A.; Ferrari, A.; Pagani, M.; Marconi, R.; et al.; "Inhibition of Candidiacidal Activity of Human Neutrophil Leukocytes by Aminoglycoside Antibiotics," *Antimicrobial Agents and Chemotherapy* pp. 87–88, Jan., 1980.

26. Belsheim, J.A.; Gnarpe, G.H.; "Antibiotics and Granulocytes; Direct and Indirect Effects on Granulocyte Chemotaxis," *Acta. Path. Mocrobiol. Scand.* Sect C, 89:217:221, 1981.

27. *Journal of Antimicrobial Chemotherapy*, 13:413, 1984.

28. Roszkowski, W.; Ko, H.L.; Toszkowski, K.; et al.; "Antibiotics and Immunomodulation: Effects of Cefotaxime, Amikacin, Mezlocillin, Piperacillin, and Clindamycin," *Med. Microbiol. Immunol.* 173:279–289, 1985.

29. Ibid.

30. Hauser, W.E.; Remington, J.S.: Effect of antibiotics on the immune response." *Am. J. Med.* 72(5):711–15, 1982.

31. Roe, D.; *Drug-Induced Nutritional Deficiencies*, AVI Publishing, Westport, Connecticut, 1976.

32. Dorfman, K.; Lemer, P.; Nadler, J.: "What puts a child at risk for developmental delays?" Presented at the Developmental Delay Registry Conference, Bethesda, Maryland, 1994.

33. Shaw, W.; Kassen, E.; Chaves, E.: "Increased Urinary Excretion of Analogs of Krebs Cycle Metabolites and Arabinose in Two Brothers with Autistic Features." *Clin. Chem.* 41(8):1094–1104, 1995.

34. Shaw, W.; Chaves, E.; Luxem, M. Abnormal Urine Organic Acids

Associated with Fungal Metabolism in Urine Samples of Children With Autism: Preliminary Results of a Clinical Trial with Antifungal Drugs. Unpublished monograph. Kansas City, Missouri, 1994.

35. Healy, G.B.; "Antimicrobial Therapy of Chronic Otitis Media with Effusion," *Int. J. Ped. Otolar.* 8:13–17, 1984.

36. Mandel, E.M.; Rockette, H.E.; Bluestone, C.D.; Paradise, J.L.; Nozza, R.J.; "Efficacy of Amoxicillin with and without Decongestant-Antihistamine for Otitis Media with Effusion in Children: Results of a Double-blind, Randomized Trial," *New Engl. J. Med.* 316:432–437, 1987.

37. Laxdal, O.E.; Merida, J.; Jones, R.H.T.: "Treatment of Acute Otitis Media: A Controlled Study of 142 Children," *Can. Med. Assoc. J.* 102:263, 1970.

38. Carlin, S.A.; et al. "Host Factors and Early Therapeutic Response in Acute Otitis Media." *J. Ped.* 118:178–83, 1991.

39. Froom, J.; et al.: "Diagnosis and Antibiotic Treatment of Acute Otitis Media: Report from the International Primary Care Network." *Br. Med. J.* 300:582–6, 1990.

40. Van Buchem, F.L.; et al.: "Therapy of Acute Otitis Media: Myringotomy, Antibiotics, or Neither? a Double-Blind Study in Children." *Lancet* 8252:883–87, 1981.

41. Van Buchem, F.L.; Peeters, M.F.; Van't Hof, M.A.: "Acute Otitis Media: A New Treatment Strategy." *Br. Med. J.* 290(6):1033–37, 1985.

42. Diamant, M.; Diamant, B.: "Abuse and Timing of Use of Antibiotics in Acute Otitis Media." *Arch. Otolaryngol.* 100:226–232, 1974.

43. Cantekin, E.I.; McGuire, T.W.; Griffith, T.L.: "Antimicrobial therapy for otitis media with effusion (secretory otitis media)." *J.A.M.A.* 266(23):3309–3317, 1991.

44. Bailar, J.: *J. Clin. Epidemiol.* 48:149–157, 1995.

45. Williams, et al.: *J.A.M.A.* 270:1344–1351, 1993.

46. Prellner, K. Personal communication with professor E. Cantekin, 1995.

47. Meistrup-Larsen, K.I.; Sorensen, H.; et al.; "Two Versus Seven Days Penicillin Treatment for Acute Otitis Media: A Placebo Controlled Trial in Children," *Acta. Otolaryngol.* 96:99–104, 1983.

48. Hendrickse, W.A.; Kusmiesz, H.; et al.; "Five vs. Ten Days of Therapy for Acute Otitis Media," *Pediatr. Infect. Dis. J.* 7:14–23, 1988.

49. Chaput de Saintonge, D.M.; Levine, D.F.; "Trial of Three-Day and Ten-Day Courses of Amoxycillin in Otitis Media," *Br. Med. J.* 284, Apr. 10, 1982.

50. Bain, J.; Murphy, E.; Ross, F.; "Acute Otitis Media: Clinical Course Among Children Who Received a Short Course of High Dose Antibiotic," *Br. Med. J.* 291, Nov. 2, 1985.

51. Van Buchem, F.L.; "Therapy of Acute Otitis Media: Myringotomy, Antibiotics, or Neither? A Double-Blind Study in Children," *Lancet* 883, Oct. 24, 1981.

52. Paparella, M.M.; Goycoolea, M.; et al.; "Silent Otitis Media: Clinical Applications," *Laryngoscope* 96:978–985, Sept., 1986.

53. Cantekin, E. The case against aggressive, expensive, and ineffective treatment of a benign disease: Comments on the clinical practice guidelines on otitis media. Feb., 1994.

54. Robson, et al. *J. Laryngol. Otol.* 1992;106:788–792.

55. Thomsen, J. Personal communication with professor E. Cantekin and Dr. Thomsen, 1995.

56. Toner, M.: "CDC—Antibiotics misused: Trend linked to increase in drug-resistant infections." *Atlanta Journal Constitution* 1995; January 18;E1.

57. Disney, F.A.: "Pediatricians, antibiotics, and office practice." *Pediatrics* 75:1135, 1984.

58. Froom J.; Culpepper, L.; et al.; "Diagnosis and Antibiotic Treatment of Acute Otitis Media: Report from International Primary Care Network," *Br. Med. J.* 300:582–6, 1990.

59. Lappé, M.; *When Antibiotics Fail: Restoring the Ecology of the Body*, North Atlantic Books, Berkeley, California, 1986.

60. Persico, M.; et al.; "Recurrent Acute Otitis Media—Prophylactic Penicillin Treatment: A Prospective Study—Part I," *Intl. J. Ped. Otolaryngol.* 10:37–46, 1985.

61. Tos, M.; Poulson, G.; Borch, J.; "Etiologic Factors in Secretory Otitis Media," *Arch. Otolaryngol.* 105(10):582–8, Oct., 1979.

62. Principi, N.; et al.; "Prophylaxis of Recurrent Acute Otitis Media and Middle Ear Effusion: Comparison of Amoxicillin with Sulfamethoxazole and Trimethoprim," *Am. J. Dis. Child.* 143:1414, Dec., 1989.

63. Lappé, M.; *When Antibiotics Fail: Restoring the Ecology of the Body*, North Atlantic Books, Berkeley, California, 1986.

64. Novick, R.P.; "Transmission of Bacterial Pathogens from Animals to Man with Special Reference to Antibiotic Resistance," *Drugs in Livestock Feed*, Vol II, Background papers, Office of Technology Assistance, pp. 3–12, June, 1979.

65. Holmberg, S.D.; Osterholm, M.T.; Senger, K.A.; Cohen, M.L.;

"Drug-Resistant Salmonella From Animals Fed Antimicrobials," *New Engl. J. Med.* 311(10): 1984.

Chapter 3. Tubes: Effectiveness, Hazards, and Complications

1. Mendelsohn, R.S.; *How to Raise a Healthy Child in Spite of Your Doctor*, Contemporary Books, Inc., Chicago, p. 134, 1984.

2. Paradise, J.L.; "On Tympanostomy Tubes; Rationale, Results, Reservations, and Recommendations," *Pediatrics* 60(1): 1977.

3. Barfold, C.; Rosborg, J.; "Secretory Otitis Media: Long-term Observations After Treatment with Grommets," *Arch. Otolaryngol.* 106:553, 1980.

4. Mawson, S.R.; "Tympanic Effusions in Childen: Long-term Results of Treatment by Myringotomy, Aspiration, and Indwelling Tubes," *J. Laryngol. Otol.* 86:105, 1972.

5. Ibid.

6. Kokko, E.; "Chronic Secretory Otitis Media in Children," *Acta. Otolaryngol.* Suppl., 327:7–44, 1974.

7. Froom, J.; "Clinical Review: Otitis Media," *J. Fam. Prac.* 15(4): 743–770, 1982.

8. Armstrong, B.W.; Armstrong, R.B.; "Chronic Non-Suppurative Otitis Media: Comparison of Tympanstomy Tubes and Medications Versus Ventilation," *Ann. Otol. Rhinol. Laryngol.* 90:533, 1981.

9. Stickler, G.B.; "The Attack on the Tympanic Membrane," *Pediatrics* Commentary, p. 291, 1984.

10. Mandel, E.M.; et al.: "Efficacy of Myringotomy With and Without Tympanostomy Tubes for Chronic Otitis Media with Effusion." *Pediatr. Infect. Dis. J.* 11:270–277, 1992.

11. Cantekin, E. The Case Against Aggressive, Expensive, and Ineffective Treatment of a Benign Disease: Comments on the Clinical Practice Guidelines on Otitis Media. Report submitted to the U.S. Congress and the Department of Health and Human Services. 50, 1994.

12. Pichichero, M.E.; Berghash, L.R; Hengerer, A.S.: "Anatomic and Audiologic Sequelae after Tympanostomy Tube Insertion or Prolonged Antibiotic Therapy for Otitis Media." *Ped. Inf. Dis. J.* 8(11):780–87, 1989.

13. Pichichero, M.E.: "Sequelae of Tympanostomy Tubes." *Ped. Inf. Dis. J.* 9(7):527–528, 1990.

14. Bodner, E.E.; Browning, G.G.; Chalmers, F.T.; Chalmers, T.C.: "Can Meta-Analysis Help Uncertainty in Surgery for Otitis Media in Children." *J. Laryngol. Otol.* 105:812–819, 1991.

15. Kleinman, L.C.; Kosecoff, J.; Dubois, R.W.; Brook, R.H.; "The Medical Appropriateness of Tympanostomy Tubes Proposed for Children Younger Than 16 Years in the United States." *J.A.M.A.* 271(16):1250–55, 1994.

16. Black, N.; Crowther, J.; Freeland, A.; "The Effectiveness of Adenoidectomy in the Treatment of Glue Ear: A Randomized Controlled Trial." *Clin. Otolaryngol.* 11:149–155, 1986.

17. Cantekin, E. The Case Against Aggressive, Expensive, and Ineffective Treatment of a benign disease: Comments on the Clinical practice guidelines on otitis media. Report submitted to the U.S. Congress and the Department of Health and Human Services. 51, 1994.

18. Sadé, J.; Luntz, M.: "Adenoidectomy in Otitis Media: A Review." *Ann. Otol. Rhinol. Laryngol.* 100:226–31, 1991.

19. Naunton, E. *Miami Herald* Nov. 29, 1988.

Chapter 4. Hearing Loss and Delayed Development: Myth or Reality?

1. Paradise, J.L.; "Otitis Media During Early Life: How Hazardous to Development? A Critical Review of the Evidence," *Pediatrics* 68(6) Dec., 1981.

2. Bluestone, C.D.; Beery, Q.C.; Paradise, J.L.; "Audiometry and Tympanometry in Relation to Middle-Ear Effusions in Children," *Laryngoscope* 83:594, 1973.

3. Mendelsohn, R.S.; "Ear Infections . . . Tubes in Ears . . . Ear Noises," *The People's Doctor* 5(5): 1985.

4. Brooks, D.N.; "Otitis Media With Effusion and Academic Attainment" *Intl. J. Ped. Otorhinolaryngol.* 12:39–47, 1986.

5. Roberts, J.E.; Sanyai, M.A.; Burchinal, M.R.; et al.; "Otitis Media in Early Childhood and its Relationship to Later Verbal and Academic Performance," *Pediatrics* 78(3) Sept., 1986.

6. Kirkwood, C.R.; Kirkwood, M.E.; "Otitis Media and Learning Disabilities: The Case for a Causal Relationship," *J. Fam. Prac.* 17(2):219–227, 1983.

7. Paradise, J.L.; "Management of Secretory Otitis Media: State of the Art," *Adv. Oto-Rhino-Laryng.* 40:99–109, 1988.

8. Paradise, J.L.; "Otitis Media During Early Life: How Hazardous to Development? A Critical Review of the Evidence," *Pediatrics* 68(6) Dec., 1981.

9. Zinkus, P.W.; Gottlieb, M.I.; Schapiro, M.; "Developmental and Psy-

choeducational Sequelae of Chronic Otitis Media," *Am. J. Dis. Child.* 132:1100, 1978.

10. Dalzell, J.; Owrid, H.L.; "Children with Conductive Deafness: A Follow-up Study," *Brit. J. Audiol.* 10:87, 1976.

11. Roberts, J.E.; Burchinal, M.R.; et al.; "Otitis Media in Early Childhood and Cognitive, Academic, and Classroom Performance of the School-Aged Child," *Pediatrics* 83(4) Apr., 1989.

12. Paradise, J.L.; "Otitis Media During Early Life: How Hazardous to Development? A Critical Review of the Evidence," *Pediatrics* 68(6) Dec., 1981.

13. Paradise, J.: *Ped. Res.,* 1993.

Chapter 5. Causes of Childhood Ear Infections

Allergy

1. Draper, W.L.; "Secretory Otitis Media," *Clinical Ecology*, Dickey, L. (Ed.), Charles Thomas, Springfield, Illinois, pp. 176–178, 1976.

2. Crook, W.G.; *Are You Allergic: A Guide to Normal Living for Allergic Adults and Children*, Professional Books, Jackson, Tennessee, 1974.

3. Draper, W.L.; "Secretory Otitis Media in Children: A Study of 540 Children," *Laryngoscope* 77:636, 1967.

4. Draper, W.L.; "The Otolaryngologist and the Allergic Child," *South. Med. J.* 59:217, 1966.

5. Bierman, C.W.; Pierson, W.E.; Donaldson, J.A.; "The Evaluation of Middle Ear Function in Children," *Am. J. Dis. Child.* 120:233–6, 1970.

6. Jordan, R.E.; "Role of Allergy in Otology," *Arch. Otolaryngol.* 55:363, 1952.

7. Derlacki, E.L.; Shambaugh, G.E., Jr.; "Allergic Management of Ear Conditions," *Trans. Am. Acad. Ophthalmol. Otolaryngol.* 57:304, 1953.

8. Pang, L.Q.; "The Importance of Allergy in Otolaryngology," *Clinical Ecology*, Dickey, L. (Ed.), Charles Thomas, Springfield, Illinois, pp. 633, 1976.

9. Heiner, D.C., "Respiratory Diseases and Food Allergy," *Ann. Allergy* 53(6 pt 2):657–64, Dec., 1984 (Review).

10. Rapp, D.; "Management of Allergy-Related Serous Otitis," *Am. J. Otol.* 5(6):463–7, Oct., 1984.

11. Shambaugh, G.E., Jr.; "Serous Otitis: Are Tubes the Answer ?" Paper presented at a meeting of the Society for Clinical Ecology and Environmental Medicine, held concurrently with the annual meeting of

the American Academy of Pediatrics (New York, Oct., 24, 1982).

12. O'Connor, R.D.; Ort, H.; Leong, A.B.; Cook, D.A.; Street, D.; Hamburger, R.N.; "Tympanometric Changes Following Nasal Antigen Challenge in Children with Allergic Rhinitis," *Ann. Allergy* 53(6):468–71, Dec., 1984.

13. Ackerman, M.N.; Friedman, R.A.; Daoyle, W.J.; Bluestone, C.D.; Fireman, P.; "Antigen-Induced Eustachian Tube Obstruction: An Intranasal Provocative Challenge Test," *J. Allergy Clin. Immunol.* 73(5 pt 1):604–9, May, 1984.

14. McGovern, J.P.; Haywood, T.J.; Fernandez, A.A.; "Allergy and Secretory Otitis Media: An Analysis of 512 Cases," *J.A.M.A.* 200:124–8, 1967.

15. Ruokonen, J.; Paganus, A.; Lehti, H.; "Elimination Diets in the Treatment of Secretory Otitis Media," *Intl. J. Ped. Otorhinolaryngol.* 4:39–46, 1982.

16. Nsouli, T.M.; et al.: "Role of Food Allergy in Serous Otitis Media." *Ann. Allergy* 73(3):215–219, 1994.

17. Bernstein, J.M.; Ellis, E.; Li, P.; "The Role of IgE-Mediated Hypersensitivity in Otitis Media With Effusion," *Otolaryngol. Head Neck Surg.* 89(5):874–8, Sept.-Oct., 1981.

18. Pastorello, E.; et al; "Evaluation of Allergic Etiology in Perennial Rhinitis," *Ann. Allergy* 55:854–56, 1985.

19. Folkers, K.; et al.; "Biochemical Evidence for a Deficiency of Vitamin B6 in Subjects Reacting to Monosodium-L-Glutamate by the Chinese Restaurant Syndrome," *Biochem. Biophys. Res. Commun.* 100:972–7, 1981.

20. Papaioannou, R.; Pfeiffer, C.C.; "Sulfite Sensitivity—Unrecognized Threat: Is Molybdenum the Cause?" *J. Orthomol. Psychiat.* 105–110, 1984.

21. Laudet, A.; Arnaud, P.; Napoly, A.; Brion, F.: The Intestinal Permeability Test Applied to the Diagnosis of Food Allergy in Pediatrics. *W.I. Med. J.* 43:87–88, 1994.

22. Speer, F.; *Food Allergy*, PSG Publishing Co. Inc., Littleton, Mass., (2nd Edition), 1983.

23. Kuvaeva, I.; "The Microecology of the Gastrointestinal Tract and the Immunological Status Under Food Allergy," *Nahrung* 28(6–7):689–93, 1984.

24. Kraemer, M.J.; Richardson, M.A.; Weiss, N.S.; Furukawa, C.T.; Shapiro, G.G.; Rierson, W.E.; Bierman, C.W.; "Risk Factors for Persistent

Middle Ear Effusions: Otitis Media, Catarrh, Cigarette Smoke Exposure, and Atopy." *J.A.M.A.*. 249(8):1022–5, Feb. 25, 1983.

25. Bonham G.S.; Wilson, R.W.; "Children's Health in Families with Cigarette Smokers," *Am. J. Publ. Hlth.* 71:290–293, 1981.

26. Ibid, pp. 290–293.

27. Pryor, W.A.; Lightsey, J.W.; Prier, D.G.; "The Production of Free Radicals *in vivo* from the Action of Xenobiotics: The Initiation of Auto-oxidation of Polyunsaturated Fatty Acids by Nitrogen Dioxide and Ozone," *Lipid Peroxides in Biology and Medicine*, New York, Academic Press, pp. 1–22, 1982.

28. National Research Council Committee on Indoor Pollutants, *Indoor Pollutants*, National Academy Press, Washington, D.C., 1981.

29. Wharton, G.W., "Mites and Commercial Extracts of House Dust" *Science* 6:1382, Mar., 1970.

30. Thatcher, R.W.; "Nutrition, Environmental Toxins and Cognitive Function," lecture, American Academy of Medical Preventics, Los Angeles, 1985.

31. Hartwell, T.D.; Zelon, H.S.; et al.; "Comparative Statistical Analysis for Volatile Halocarbons in Indoor and Outdoor Air," *Indoor Air*, 4:57–62, Swedish Council for Building Research, Stockholm, Sweden, 1984.

32. Rosenweig, M.; Hartwell, T.D.; " Statistical Analysis and Evaluation of the Halocarbon Survey," Research Triangle Institute, Final Report, EPA Contract; 68–01-5848, 1983.

33. Wallace, L.; Pellizzari, E.; et al.; "Exposure to Volatile Organic Compounds: Direct Measurement in Breathing-Zone Air, Drinking Water, Food, and Exhaled Breath," *Env. Res.* 35:193–211, 1984.

34. Gammage, R.B.; White, D.A.; Gupta, K.C.; "Residential Measurements of High Volatility Organics and Their Sources," *Indoor Air* 4:157–162, Swedish Council for Building Research, Stockholm, Sweden, 1984.

35. Molhave, L.; Moller, J.; "The Atmospheric Environment in Modern Danish Dwellings: Measurements in 39 Flats," *Indoor Climate*, pp. 171–186, Danish Building Research Institute, Copenhagen, 1979.

36. Jarke, F.J.; *ASHRAE Rp 183*, IITRI, Chicago, 1979.

37. Lebret, E.; Van de Wiel, A.; et al.; "Volatile Hydrocarbons in Dutch Homes," *Indoor Air* 4:169–174, Swedish Council for Building Research, Stockholm, Sweden, 1984.

38. Seifert, B.; Abraham, H.J.; "Indoor Air Concentrations of Benzene

and Some Other Aromatic Hydrocarbons," *Ecotoxicol. Env. Safety* 6:190–192 1982.

39. Gammage, R.B.; Kaye, S.V.; *Indoor Air and Human Health,* 2nd printing, Lewis Publishers, Chelsea, Michigan, 1985.

40. Ibid.

41. Molhave, L.; "The Relation Between Emission Rate of Organic Gases, etc, from Building Materials and Their Concentrations in the Indoor Environment," *6th World Congress on Air Quality.* 2:345–352, Paris, 1983.

42. Sterling, D.A.; "Volatile Organic Compounds in Indoor Air: An Overview of Sources, Concentrations, and Health Effects," *Indoor Air and Human Health,* ed. by Gammage, R.B., and Kaye, S.V., Lewis Publishers, Inc., Chelsea, MI, 1984.

Infection

43. Froom, J.; "Otitis Media: Clinical Review," *J. Fam. Pract.* 15(4):743–770, 1982.

44. Howie, V.M.; Ploussard, J.H.; Lester, R.L.; "Otitis Media: A Clinical and Bacteriological Correlation," *Pediatrics* 45:29, 1970.

45. Klein, J.O.; "Microbiology of Otitis Media," *Ann. Otol. Rhinol. Laryngol.* 89 (Suppl. 68):98, 1980.

46. Asman, B.J.; Fireman, P.; "The Role of Allergies in the Development of Otitis Media with Effusion," *Intl. Ped.* 3(3): July-Sept., 1988.

47. Stephenson, A.; et al.: Proceedings of the 5th International Symposium on Otitis Media, 389–392, 1993.

48. Renvall, J, et al.: Proceedings of the 4th International Symposium on Otitis Media, 326–328, 1988.

49. Post, J.C.; et al.: "Molecular Analysis of Bacterial Pathogens in Otitis Media with Effusion." *J.A.M.A.* 273:1598–1604, 1995.

50. Chonmaitree, T.; et al.: "Effect of Viral Respiratory Tract Infection on Outcome of Acute Otitis Media." *J. Pediatr.* 120:856–862, 1992.

51. Cohen, S.R.; Thompson, J.W.: "Otitic Candidiasis in Children: Evaluation of the Problem and Effectiveness of Ketoconazole in 10 Patients." *Ann. Otol. Rhinol. Laryngol.* 99:427–431, 1990.

52. Klein, J.O.; "Microbiology of Otitis Media," *Ann. Otol. Rhinol. Laryngol.* 89 (Suppl. 68):98, 1980.

53. Asman, B.J.; Fireman, P.; "The Role of Allergies in the Development of Otitis Media with Effusion," *Intl. Ped.* 3(3): July-Sept., 1988.

54. Pelton, S.I.; Teele, D.W.; Shurin, P.A.; et al.; "Disparate Cultures

of Middle Ear Fluids," *Am. J. Dis. Child.* 134:951, 1980.

55. Schwartz, R.; Rodriguez, W.; et al.; "The Increasing Incidence of Ampicillin-Resistant *Haemophilus influenzae:* A Cause of Otitis Media," *J.A.M.A.* 239(4): Jan. 23, 1978.

56. Chandra, R.K.; "Trace Element Regulation of Immunity and Infection," *Am. J. Clin. Nutr.* 35:417–68 (Suppl.), 1985.

57. Bondestam, M.; Foucard, T.; Gebre-Medhin, M.; "Subclinical Trace Element Deficiency in Children with Undue Susceptibility to Infections," *Act. Paed. Sc.* 74:515–520, 1985.

58. Golden, M.; Jackson, A.; Golden, B.; "Effect of Zinc on Thymus of Recently Malnourished Children," *Lancet,* ii:1057–9, 1977.

59. Beisel, W.R.; "Single Nutrients and Immunity," *Am. J. Clin. Nutr.* 35:417–68 (Suppl.), 1982.

60. Werbach, M.R.; Nutritional Influences on Illness: *A Sourcebook of Clinical Research,* Third Line Press, Inc., Tarzana, CA, p. 252, 1987.

61. Beach, R.; Gershwin, M.; Hurley, L.; "Persistent Immunological Consequences of Gestational Zinc Deprivation," *Am. J. Clin. Nutr.* 38:579–90, 1983.

62. Sanchez, A.; et al.; "Role of Sugars in Human Neutrophilic Phagocytosis," *Am. J. Clin. Nutr.* 26:180, 1973.

63. Lewis, M.; et al.: Prenatal Exposure to Heavy Metals: Effect on Childhood Cognitive Skills and Health Status. *Pediatrics* 89:1010–1015, 1992.

64. Shannon, M.W.; Graef, J.W.: "Lead Intoxication in Infancy." *Pediatrics* 89(1):87–90, 1992.

Mechanical Obstruction

65. Ford, F.R.; "Breech Delivery in its Possible Relations to Injury of the Spinal Cord with Special Reference to Infantile Paraplegia," *Arch. Neurol. Psychiat.* 14:742, 1925.

66. Towbin, A.; "Latent Spinal Cord and Brain Stem Injury in Newborn Infants," *Develop. Med. Child. Neurol.* 11:54–68, 1969.

67. Duncan, J.M.; "Laboratory Note: On the Tensile Strength of the Fresh Adult Foetus," *Brit. Med. J.* ii:763, 1874.

68. Frymann, V.; "Relations of Disturbances of Cranio-sacral Mechanisms to Symptomatology of the Newborn," *J. Am. Osteopathic Assoc.* 65:1059, 1966.

69. Degenhardt, B.F.; Kuchera, M.L.: The Prevalence of Cranial Dysfunction in Children with a History of Otitis Media from Kindergarten

to Third Grade. Kirksville College of Osteopathic Medicine, Kirksville, Missouri. Unpublished mongraph.

70. Youniss, S.: The Relationship Between Craniomandibular Disorders and Otitis Media in Children. *J. Craniomandib. Pract.* 9(2):169–73, 1991.

71. Replace ref 73 with: Grosfeld, O, Czarnecka, B. "Musculo-Articular Disorders of the Stomatognathic System in School Children Examined According to Clinical Criteria." *J. Oral Rehabil.* 4:193–200, 1977.

72. replace ref. 74 with: Wanman, A.; Agerberg, G.; "Two Year Longitudinal Study of Signs of Mandibular Dysfunction in Adolescents." *Acta. Odontal. Scand.* 44:333–342, 1986.

73. Bean, M. Part of a lecture on TMJ dysfunction, Baltimore, MD, 1984

74. Marasa, F.; Ham, B.; "Case Reports Involving the Treatment of Children with Chronic Otitis Media with Effusion Via Craniomandibular Methods." *J. Craniomandib.* Pract. 6:256–270, 1988.

75. Upledger, J.: Craniosacral Therapy. Seattle: Eastland Press, 1983.

76. Gutmann, G.; "Das Atlas-Blockierungs-Syndrome des Sauglings und des Kleinkindes," *Manuelle Med.* 25:5–10, 1987.

77. Peters, R.E.; Chance, M.E.; "A Priceless Legacy-Lost, Strayed or Forfeited?" *J. Austral. Chiropr. Assoc.* 18(3):81–84, Sept., 1988.

78. Chapman-Smith, D.; "Blocked Atlantal Nerve Syndrome in Babies and Infants," *The Chiropractic Report* 3, 2., Jan. 1989 (a review of Peters & Chance, and Gutmann is provided).

Nutrient Insufficiency

79. Rudin, D.O.; "Omega-3 Essential Fatty Acids in Medicine," *1984–1985 Yearbook of Nutritional Medicine,* Bland, J.S. (Ed.), Keats Publishing, New Canaan, Connecticut, p. 41, 1985.

80. Ibid, p. 42.

81. Rudin, D.O.; Felix, C.; *The Omega-3 Phenomenon,* Avon Books, New York, 1987.

82. Holman, R.T.; Johnson, S.B.; Ogburn, P.L.: "Deficiency of Essential Fatty Acids and Membrane Fluidity During Pregnancy and Lactation." *Proc. Nat. Acad. Sci.* 88:4835–4839, 1991.

83. Rudin, D.O.; Felix, C.; *The Omega-3 Phenomenon,* Avon Books, New York, 1987, p. 22.

84. Moser, P.; Reynolds, R.; "Dietary Zinc Intake and Zinc Concentrations of Plasma, Erythrocytes, and Breastmilk in Antepartum and

Postpartum Lactating and Non-Lactating Women: A Longitudinal Study," *Am. J. Clin. Nut.* 38:101–108, 1983.

85. Grandgirard, A.; et al.: "Incorporation of Trans Long-Chain n-3 Polyunsaturated Fatty Acids in Rat Brain Structures and Retina" *Lipids* 29(4):251–258, 1994.

86. Holman, R.T.; Johnson, S.; Hatch, T.F.; "A Case of Human Linolenic Acid Deficiency Involving Neurological Abnormalities," *Am. J. Clin. Nutr.* 35:617–23, 1982.

87. Enig, M.G.; Pallansch, L.A.; Sampugna, J.; Keeney, M.; "Fatty Acid Composition of the Fat in Selected Food Items With Emphasis on Trans Components," *J. Am. Oil Chem. Soc.* 60:1788–1795, 1983.

88. "Trans Fatty Acids in Foods," *Nutrition Reviews* 42(8): 1984.

89. Erasmus, U.; *Fats and Oils: The Complete Guide to Fats and Oils in Health and Nutrition*, Alive Books, Vancouver, Canada, 1986.

90. "Trans Fatty Acids in Foods," *Nutrition Reviews* 42(8): 1984.

91. Enig, M.G.; Pallansch, L.A.; Sampugna, J.; Keeney, M.; "Fatty Acid Composition of the Fat in Selected Food Items With Emphasis on Trans Components," *J. Am. Oil Chem. Soc.* 60:1788–1795, 1983.

92. Enig, M.G.; Subodh, A.; Keeney, M.; Sampugna, J.: "Isomeric Trans Fatty Acids in the U.S. Diet." *J. Am. Col. Nutr.* 9(5):471–486, 1990.

93. Horrobin, D.F.; "Essential Fatty Acids: A Review," in *Clinical Uses of Essential Fatty Acids*, Eden Press, New York, pp. 3–31, 1982.

94. Berkson, D.; "Nutritional Considerations for Female Health Problems," lecture on clinical nutrition presented in Bloomington, Minnesota, Nov., 1987.

95. Ibid.

96. Rudin, D.O.; "Omega-3 Essential Fatty Acids in Medicine," *1984–1985 Yearbook of Nutritional Medicine*, Bland, JS (Ed.), Keats Publishing, New Canaan, Connecticut, p. 41, 1985.

97. Pennington, J.A.T.; Young, B.E.; et al.; "Mineral Content of Foods and Total Diets: The Selected Minerals in Foods Survey, 1982 to 1984," Food and Drug Administration, Kansas City, Missouri.

98. Bendich, A.; "Vitamin E status of U.S. children." *J. Am. Col. Nutr.* 11(4):441–44, 1992.

99. Controlled Trial on the use of Oral N-acetylcysteine in the Treatment of Glue-Ear Following Drainage. *European J Respir Dis* 61 (Supplement 111):158, 1980.

100. Chole, R.A.; "Squamous Metaplasia of the Middle Ear Mucosa During Vitamin A Deprivation," *Otolaryngol. Head Neck Surg.* 87(6):837–44,

Nov.-Dec., 1979.

101. Golden, M.; Jackson, A.; Golden, B.; "Effect of Zinc on Thymus of Recently Malnourished Children," *Lancet* ii:1057–9, 1977.

102. Bondestam, M.; Foucard, T.; Gebre-Medhin, M.; "Subclinical Trace Element Deficiency in Children with Undue Susceptibility to Infections," *Act. Paed. Sc.* 74:515–520, 1985.

103. Manku, M.S.; et al.; "Reduced Levels of Prostaglandin Precursors in the Blood of Atopic Patients: Defective Delta-6-Desaturase Function as a Biochemical Basis for Atopy," *Prostaglandins, Leukotrienes in Medicine* 9:615–28, 1982.

104. Galland, L.; "Increased Requirements for Essential Fatty Acids in Atopic Individuals: A Review with Clinical Descriptions," *J. Am. Col. Nutr.* 5:213–28, 1986.

105. Skoner, D.P.; Stillwagon, P.K.; et al.; "Inflammatory Mediators in Chronic Otitis Media with Effusion," *Arch. Otolaryngol. Head Neck Surg.* 114:1131–1133, Oct. 1988.

106. Jung, T.T.K.; "Prostaglandins, Leukotrienes, and Other Arachidonic Acid Metabolites in the Pathogenesis of Otitis Media," *Laryngoscope* 98: Sept. 1988.

107. Stenmark, K.R.; James, S.L.; et al.; "Leukotriene C4 and D4 in Neonates with Hypoxemia and Pulmonary Hypertension," *New Engl. J. Med.* 309:77, 1983.

108. Goldman, D.W.; Goetzl, E.J.; "Mediation and Modulation of Immediate Hypersensitivity and Inflammation by Products of the Oxygenation of Arachidonic Acid," *Immunology of Inflammation*, P.A. Ward, (Ed.) Elsevier Science Pub., New York, pp. 163–187, 1976.

109. Dahlen, S.; Sammuelsson, B.; "Leukotrienes are Potent Constrictors of Human Bronchi," *Nature* 288:484, 1980.

110. Hanna, C.J.; Bach, M.K.; et al.; "Slow-reacting Leukotrienes and Pulmonary Vascular Smooth Muscle in vitro," *Nature* 210:343,1981.

111. Jung, T.T.K.; "Prostaglandins, Leukotrienes, and Other Arachidonic Acid Metabolites in the Pathogenesis of Otitis Media," *Laryngoscope* 98: Sept. 1988.

112. Smith, D.M.; Jung, T.T.K.; Juhn, S.K.; Berlinger, N.T.; Gerrard, J.M.; "Prostaglandins in Experimental Otitis Media," *Arch. Otorhinolaryngol.* 225:207–9, 1979.

113. Skoner, D.P.; Stillwagon, P.K.; et al.; "Inflammatory Mediators in Chronic Otitis Media with Effusion," *Arch. Otolaryngol. Head Neck Surg.* 114:1131–1133, Oct. 1988.

114. Jung, T.T.K.; Giebink, G.S.; Juhn, S.K.; "Effects of Ibuprofen, Corticosteroid, Penicillin on the Pathogenesis of Experimental Pneumococcal Otitis Media," *Recent Advances in Otitis Media with Effusion*, D.J. Lim, C.D. Bluestone, J.O. Klein, et al. (Eds.), BC Decker, Inc., Philadelphia, pp. 269–272, 1984.

115. Roe, D.; Drug-Induced Nutritional Deficiency, AVI Publishing Co., Westport, Connecticut, 1976.

116. Stool, S.; et al.: "Otitis Media with Effusion." U.S. Department of Health and Human Services, AHCPR Publication No. 94-0622, 1994.

Chapter 6 Home Care for Earaches

1. Wootan, G.; "Home-Care for Children," *Mothering* Winter, p. 38, 1985.

2. Moskowitz, R.; "Unvaccinated Children," *Mothering* Winter, 1987.

3. Cummings, S.; Ullman, D.; *Everybody's Guide to Homeopathic Medicines*, Jeremy P. Tarcher, Los Angeles, p. 113, 1984.

4. Thompson, L.L.; "Fear of Fever is Often Worse Than Fever Itself," *Washington Post* review reprinted in the *Minneapolis Star Tribune* Nov. 10, 1989.

5. Nelson, K.B.; Ellenberg, J.H.; "Prognosis in Children with Febrile Seizures," *Pediatrics* May, 1978; Schmitt, B. D.; "Fever Phobia," *Am. J. Dis. of Child.* 176–186, Feb. 1980.

6. Mendelsohn, R.S.; *How to Raise a Healthy Child in Spite of Your Doctor*, Contemporary Books, Inc., Chicago, pp. 66–79, 1984.

7. Carmichael, L.E.; Barnes, F.D.; Percy, D.H.; "Temperature as a Factor in Resistance of Young Puppies," *J. Infect. Dis.* 120:669, 1969.

8. Kluger, M.J.; "Fever," *Pediatrics* 66:720–724, 1980.

9. Kluger, M.J.; Rothenberg, B.A.; "Fever and Reduced Iron: Their Interaction as a Host Defense Response to Bacterial Infection," *Science* 203:374, 1979.

10. Schmitt, B.D.; "Fever Phobia," *Am. J. Dis. Child.* 176–186, Feb., 1980.

11. Nelson, K.B.; Ellenberg, J.H.; "Prognosis in Children with Febrile Seizures," *Pediatrics* May, 1978.

12. Mendelsohn, R.S.; *How to Raise a Healthy Child in Spite of Your Doctor*, Contemporary Books, Inc., Chicago, pp. 75, 1984.

13. Replace reference 13 with: Jaffe, D.M.: "High Fever: is Early Antibiotic Treatment Useful?" *N. Engl. J. Med.* 317:1175, 1987.

14. Doran, T.F.; DeAngelis, C.; Baumgardner, R.A.; Mellitis, E.D.;

"Acetaminophen: More Harm Than Good for Chickenpox?" *J. Pediatrics* 114(6):1045–8, 1989.

15. Mendelsohn, R.S.; *How to Raise a Healthy Child in Spite of Your Doctor,* Contemporary Books, Inc., Chicago, pp. 78–79, 1984.

16. Meduski, J.W.; *Practical Guidelines for the Selection and Application of Lactobacilli and Bifidobacteria in Preventive Medicine and Therapy,* unpublished guidelines, 1988.

17. Boyce, T.W., et al.: "Influence of Life Events and Family Routines on Childhood Respiratory Tract Illness." *Pediatrics* 60(4):609–615, 1977.

18. Meyer, R.J.; Haggerty, R.J.: "Streptococcal Infections in Families." *Pediatrics* 4:539–49, 1962.

19. Bjorkstein, B.; Back, O.; Gustavson, K.; et al.; "Zinc and Immune Function in Down's Syndrome," *Acta. Paediatr. Scand.* 69:183–187, 1980.

20. "Correction of Impaired Immunity in Down's Syndrome by Zinc," *Nutrition Reviews* 38:11:365–7, 1980.

21. Anneren, G.; Magnusson, C.G.M.; Nordvall, S.L.: "Increase in Serum Concentrations of IgG2 and IgG4 by Selenium Supplementation in Children with Down's Syndrome." *Arch. Dis. Child.* 65:1353–55, 1990.

22. Thomas, C. Personal communication, 1995.

23. Bralley, J.A.: Personal communication, 1995.

24. Rowe, A.H.; *Clinical Allergy,* Philadelphia, Lea and Febiger, 1937.

25. Crook W.G.; *The Yeast Connection,* Professional Books, Jackson, Tennessee, pp. 18–26, 1985.

26. Ibid, p. 77.

27. Florey, H.W.; *British Medical Journal* 654, 1943.

28. Chedid, L.; Parent, M.; Boyer, F.; Skarnes, R.C.; "Non-Specific Host Response in Tolerance to the Lethal Effect of Endotoxin," *Bacterial Endotoxins,* M. Landy and W. Braun, (eds.), Rutgers, the State University, p. 112, 1964.

29. Boswinkel, J.C.; The effects of homeopathic dilutions of DDVP on locusts in the Northwestern Sahara, Personal communication, 1989.

30. Riley, D.T.; Taylor, M.A.; "Is Homeopathy a Placebo Response: Controlled Trial of Homeopathic Potency, with Pollen in Hayfever as Model," *Lancet* 881–886, Oct. 18, 1986.

31. Moessinger, P.; "Zur Behandlung der Otitis Media mit Pulsatilla," *Allgemeine Homoopathische Zeitung* 230:89, 1985.

32. Neustaedter, R.; "Management of Otitis Media with Effusion in Homoeopathic Practice," *J. Am. Inst. Homeop.* 79(3, 4) 1986.

33. Reilly, D.T.; et al.: "Is Evidence for Homeopathy Reproducible?"

Lancet 344:1601–1606, 1994.

34. Cummings, S.; Ullman, D.; *Everybody's Guide to Homeopathic Medicines,* Jeremy P. Tarcher, Los Angeles, pp. 41–42, 1984.

35. Chapman-Smith, D.; "Blocked Atlantal Nerve Syndrome in Babies and Infants," *The Chiropractic Report,* Jan. 1989, 3(2) (a review of Peters & Chance and Gutmann is provided).

36. Gutmann, G.; "Das Atlas-Blockierungs-Syndrome des Sauglings und des Kleinkindes," *Manuelle Med.* 25:5–10, 1987.

37. Hoffman, D.; *The Holistic Herbal,* The Findhorn Press, Findhorn, Moray, Scotland, 1983.

38. Meruelo, D.; et al.; *Proceedings of the National Academy of Sciences,* 85:5230–4, July 1988.

39. *The Biology and Cultivation of Edible Mushrooms,* Chang and Hayes, (eds.), Academic Press, Inc., pp. 169–187, 1978.

40. Salmi, H.A.; Sarne, S.; *Effects of Silymarin on Chemical, Functional, and Morphological Alterations of the Liver: A Double-Blind, Placebo-Controlled Study,* Central Military Hospital-1, Dept. of Public Health, Helsinki, Finland, Sept. 25 1981.

41. Ikeda, K.; Takasaka, T.; "Treatment of Secretory Otitis Media with Kampo Medicine," *Arch. Otorhinolaryngol.* 245:234–236, 1988.

42. Benedict, M.; Personal communication, 1989.

43. "Echinacea," *Medical Nutrition* 4(2):14–16, 1989.

44. Rasic, J.L.; Kurman, J.A.; *Bifidobacteria and Their Role,* Birkhauser Verlag, Basel-Boston-Stuttgart, 1983.

45. Speck, P.; Gilliand, A.; "Antagonistic Action of L. Acidophilus Toward Intestinal and Foodborne Pathogens in Associative Cultures," *J. Food Prot.* 40(12):820–823, 1977.

46. Shahani, K.M.; Hathaway, I.L.; and Kelly, P.L.; "B-complex Vitamin Content of Cheese. II Niacin, Pantothenic Acid, Pyridoxine, Biotin & Folic Acid," *J. Dairy Sci.* 45:833, 1962

47. Shahani, K.M.; Kilara, A.; "Lactase Activity of Cultured and Acidified Dairy Products," *J. Dairy Sci.* 59:2031, 1976.

48. Dubos, R.; *The Microbiota In Man Adapting,* Yale University Press, New Haven, Connecticut, p. 110, 1965.

49. Goldin, B.; Gorbach, S.L.; "Alterations in Fecal Microflora Enzymes Related to Age, Lactobacili Supplements and Dimethyl Hydrazine," *Cancer* 40:2421, 1977.

50. Ibid.

51. Friend, B.A.; Rarmer, R.E.; Shahani, K.M.; "Effect of Feeding and

Intraperitoneal Implantation of Yogurt Culture Cells on Ehrlich Ascites Tumor." *Milchwissenschaff* 37 (12), 1982.

52. Purohit, B.C.; Joshi, K.P.; et al.; "The formation of Germtubes by Candida albicans, when Grown with Staphylococcus pyogenes, E. coli, Klebsiella pneumoniae, L. acidophilus and Proteus vulgaris," *Mycopathologia* 62 (3):187–189, 1977.

53. Mayer, J.B.; "Viren Und Darmflora," *Paediat. Paedol* 1:131–137, 1965.

54. Meduski, J.W.; *Practical Guidelines for the Selection and Application of Lactobacilli and Bifidobacteria in Preventive Medicine and Therapy,* unpublished guidelines, 1988.

Chapter 7 Preventing Ear Infections in Your Child

1. Chandra, R.K.; "Prospective Studies of the Effect of Breastfeeding on Incidence of Infection and Allergy," *Acta. Pediatr. Scand.* 68(5):691–4, 1979.

2. Ibid.

3. Ibid.

4. Saarinen, U.; "Breastfeeding Prevents Otitis Media," *Nutrition Reviews* 41(8):241, 1983.

5. Sassen, M.L.; Brand, R.; Grote, J.J.: "Breast-feeding and Acute Otitis Media." *Am. J. Otolaryngol.* 15(5):351–357, 1994.

6. Paradise, J.L.; Elster, B.A.; Tan, L.: "Evidence in Infants with Cleft Palate that Breast Milk Protects Against Otitis Media." *Pediatrics* 94(6 Pt 1):853–860, 1994.

7. Hanson, L.A.; et al.: "Breast Feeding: Overview and Breast Milk Immunology." *Acta. Paediatr. Jpn.* 36(5):557–561, 1994.

8. Birch, E.; et al. "Breast-feeding and Optimal Visual Development." *J. Pediatr. Opthalmol. Strabismus* 30(1):33–38, 1993.

9. Lucas, A.; Morley, R.; Cole, T.J.; Lister, G.; Leeson-Payne.: "Breast Milk and Subsequent Intelligence Quotient in Children Born Preterm." *Lancet* 239:261–264, 1992.

10. Gammage, R.B.; Kaye, S.V.; *Indoor Air and Human Health,* 2nd printing, Lewis Publishers, Chelsea, Michigan, 1985.

11. Kenny, E.; New York Research Laboratory, memo, 1985.

12. Minnesota Department of Health, memo, 1989.

13. Wald, E.R.; Dashefsky, B.; et al.; "Frequency and Severity of Infections in Day Care," *J. Pediatr.* 112:540–6, 1988.

14. Pickering, L.K.; Woodward, W.E.; "Diarrhea in Day Care Centers," *Ped. Infect. Dis. J.* 1(1):47–51, 1982.

15. Schuman, S.; "Day Care Associated Infection: More Than Meets the Eye," *J.A.M.A.* Jan. 7, 1983.

16. Redmond, S.; Pichichero, M.; "*Haemophilus influenzae* Type b Disease: An Epidemiologic Study with Special Reference to Day Care Centers," *J.A.M.A.* 252(18):2581–2584, 1984.

17. Black, R.E.; Dykes, A.C.; Sinclair, S.P.; Wells, J.G.; "Giardiasis in Day-Care Centers: Evidence of Person-to-Person Transmission," *Pediatrics* 60(4): 1977.

18. Jasper, W.F.; "My Mother the State: But is it Good for Kids?" *The New American* 5(3): 1989.

19. Johnson, A.S.; Leibowitz, A.; Waite, L.J.; "Child Care and Children's Illness," *Am. J. Pub. Hlth.* 78(9):1175–1177, 1988.

20. Wald, E.R.; Dashefsky, B.; et al.; "Frequency and Severity of Infections in Day Care," *J. Pediatr.* 112:540–6, 1988.

21. Strangert, K.; "Otitis media in Young Children in Different Types of Day Care," *Scand. J. Infect. Dis.* 9:119–23, 1977.

22. Pukander, J.; Sipila, M.; Karma, P.; "Occurrence of and Risk Factors in Acute Otitis Media. In: Lim D.J., Bluestone, D.C., Klein, J.O., Nelson, J.D., eds. *Recent Advances in Otitis Media With Effusion,* B C Decker, Philadelphia, pp. 9–13, 1984.

23. Birch, L.; Elbrond, O.; "Prospective Epidemiological Study of Secretory Otitis Media in Chilren not Attending Kindergarten, An Incidence Study," *Intl. J. Ped. Otorhinolaryngol.* 11:183–190, 1986.

24. Wald, E. R.; Dashefsky, B.; et al.; "Frequency and Severity of Infections in Day Care," *J. Pediatr.* 112:540–6, 1988.

25. Benedict, M.; Personal Communication, 1989.

26. Bolton-Smith, C.; Woodward, M.: "Antioxidant Vitamin Adequacy in Relation to Consumption of Sugars." *Eur. J. Clin. Nutr.* 49:124–133, 1995.

27. Cheraskin, E.; "Sucrose, Neutrophilic Phagocytosis and Resistance to Disease," *Dental Survey* 52(12):46–48, 1976.

28. Durlack, J.; *Le Diabete* 19:99–113, 1971.

29. Lindeman, R.D.; et al.; *Magnesium in Health and Disease,* SP Medical and Scientific Books, Jamaica, NY, pp. 236–45, 1980.

30. Freundlich, M.; et al.; "Infant Formula as a Cause of Aluminum Toxicity in Neonatal Uremia," *Lancet* 2:527–29, 1985.

31. Pesce; McKean; "Toxic Susceptibilities in the Newborn with Special Consideration with Polysorbate Toxicity," *Ann. Clin. Lab. Sci.* 19:70–73, 1989.

32. "Plasma Aluminum Measurements in Term Infants Fed Human Milk or a Soy-Based Infant Formula," *Pediatrics* 84(6): 1105–7, Dec., 1989.

33. Kozlovsky, A.S.; et al.; "Effects of Diets High in Simple Sugars on Urinary Chromium Losses," *Metabolism* 35:515–18, 1986.

34. Flaws, B.; "Stagnant Food and Pediatric Disease: The Care and Feeding of Infants According to Traditional Chinese Medicine," *Am. J. Acupunct.* 17(4):331–336, 1989.

Chapter 8. Alternative Treatment: Some Solutions

1. Akerle, O.; "The Best of Both Worlds: Bringing Traditional Medicine up to Date," *Soc. Sci. Med.* 24(2):177–181, 1987.

2. Eisenberg, L.; "Preventive Pediatrics: The Promise and the Peril," *Pediatrics* 80(3):415–416, 1987.

3. Ikeda, K.; Takasaka, T.; "Treatment of Secretory Otitis Media with Kampo Medicine," *Arch. Oto-Rhino-Laryngol.* 245:234–236, 1988.

4. Lildholdt, T.; "Unilateral Grommet Insertion and Adenoidectomy in Bilateral Secretory Otitis Media: Preliminary Report of the Results in 91 Children," *Clin. Otolaryngol.* 4:87–93, 1982. The quote appears in a footnote to this paper.

5. Paparella, M.M.; "Complications and Sequelae of Otitis Media: State of the Art," in Lim, D.J. (ed.) *Recent Advances in Otitis Media with Effusion,* B.C. Decker, Inc., Burlingtion, Ontario, Canada, pp. 316–319, 1984.

6. Levine, S.A.; Kidd, P.M.; *Antioxidant Biochemical Adaptation: Doorways to the New Science and Medicine,* Biocurrents Research Corporation, San Francisco, 1984.

7. Bland, J.S.; Baker, S.M.; *Immune Modulation: The Prevention of Immunosenscence,* HealthComm, Inc., Gig Harbor, WA, 1989.

8. Messer, S.; *Homeopathy & Otitis in Children,* Audio Taped Lecture, Homeopathic Educational Services, Berkeley, California, 1986.

9. Ibid.

10. Ibid.

11. Borland, D.M.; *Children's Types,* World Homeopathic Links, New Dehli-110055.

12. Santwani, M.T.; *Common Ailments of Children and Their Homeopathic Management,* Jain Publishing Co., New Delhi, 1983.

13. Neustaedter, R.; "Management of Otitis Media with Effusion in Homeopathic Practice," *J. Am. Inst. Homeop.* 79(3, 4):19, 1986.

14. Houghton, H.C.; *Lectures on Clinical Otology,* Otis Clapp & Son, New York Homeopathic Medical College, 1885.

15. Gutmann, G.; and Medizin, M.; "Blocked Atlantal Nerve Syndrome in Babies and Infants," *Manual Med.* 25:5–10, 1987.

16. La Francis, M.E.; "A Chiropractic Perspective on Atlantoaxial Instability in Down's Syndrome," *J. Manip. Phys. Therap.* March/ April, 1990. (*See also,* Davidson, R. G.; "Atlantoaxial Instability in Individuals with Down Syndrome: A Fresh Look at the Evidence," *Pediatrics* 81(6) 1988.

17. Scott, J.; "The Treatment of Children by Acupuncture," *The Journal of Chinese Medicine,* England, 1986.

18. *Essentials of Chinese Acupuncture,* Foreign Languages Press, Beijing, 1980.

19. Becker, R.O.; *Cross Currents: The Perils of Electropollution, The Promise of Electromedicine,* Jeremy P. Tarcher, Inc., Los Angeles, pp. 130–132, 1990.

20. White, A.; Personal communication, 1990.

21. Benedict, M.; Personal communication, 1989.

22. Jung, T.T.K.; "Prostaglandins, Leukotrienes, and Other Arachidonic Acid Metabolites in the Pathogenesis of Otitis Media," *Laryngoscope* 98:983, 1988.

23. *Proceedings of the National Academy of Sciences* 86(16): 1989. Includes a discussion of Ascorbic acid as a free-radical scavenger.

24. Loh, H. S.; Walters, K.; Wilson, C.W. M.; "The Effects of Aspirin on the Metabolic Availability of Ascorbic Acid in Detoxification of Human Beings," *J. Clin. Pharmacol.* 13:480, 1973.

25. Nandi, B.K.; Subramanian, N.; Majumder, A.k.; Chatterjee, I.B.; "Effect of Ascorbic Acid on Detoxification of Histamine Under Stress Conditions," *Biochem. Pharm.* 23:643–647, 1974.

26. Hausteen, B.; "Flavonoids, a Class of Natural Products of High Pharmacologic Potency," *Biochem. Pharm.* 32:(7):1141–1148, 1983.

27. Voorhees, J.J.; "Leukotrienes and Other Lipoxygenase Products in the Pathogenesis and Therapy of Psoriasis and Other Dermatoses," *Arch. Dermatol.* 119:541–547, 1983.

28. Srimal, R.C.; Dhawan, B.N.; "Pharmacology of Diferuloyo Methane (Curcumin), a Non-Steroidal Anti-Inflammatory Agent," *J. Pharm. Pharmac.* 25:447–452.

29. Chandra, D.; Gupta, S.S.; "Anti-Inflammatory and Anti-Arthritic Activity of Volatile Oil of *Curcuma longa,*" *Indian J. Med. Res.* 60:138–142, 1972.

30. Sharma, S.C.; Mukhtar, H.; et al.; "Lipid Peroxide Formation in Experimental Inflammation," *Biochem. Pharm.* 21:1210–1214, 1972.

31. Salimath, B.P.; Sundaresh, C.S.; Srinivas, L.; "Dietary Components Inhibit Lipid Peroxidation in Erythrocyte Membrane," *Nutr. Res.* 6:1171–1178, 1986.

32. Bauman, J.; Wrun, G.; et al.; "Effect of Quercitin on Prostaglandin Synthetase," *Prosataglandins* 20:627, 1980.

33. Underhill, J.; "Bioflavonoids—Chemistry and Physiology," *Can. J. Biochem. Physiol.* 35:219, 1957.

34. Regtop, H.; "Nutriton, Leukotrienes and Inflammatory Disorders," *1984–85 Yearbook of Nutritional Medicine,* J. Bland (ed.), Keats Publishing, Inc., New Canaan, Connecticut, pp. 55–69, 1985.

35. Flynn, D.L.; et al.; "Inhibition of Human Neutrophil 5-Lipoxygenase Activity by Gingerdione, Shogaoi, Capsaicin and Related Pungent Compounds," *Prost. Leuk. Med.* 24:195–198, 1986.

36. Ikeda, K.; Takasaka, T.; "Treatment of Secretory Otitis Media with Kampo Medicine," *Arch. Oto-Rhino-Laryngol.* 245:234–236, 1988.

37. Gilbert, V.A.; Zebrowski, E.J.; Chan, A.C.; "Differential Effects of Megavitamin E on Prostaglandin and Thromboxane Synthesis in Streptozotocin-Induced Diabetic Rats," *Horm. Metabol. Res.* 15:320–325, 1983.

38. Voorhees, J.J.; "Leukotrienes and Other Lipoxygenase Products in the Pathogenesis and Therapy of Psoriasis and Other Dermatoses," *Arch. Dermatol.* 119:541–547, 1983.

39. Chandra, R.K.; "Sinlge Nutrient Deficiency and Cell-Mediated Immunity: Zinc," *Amer. J. Clin. Nutr.* 33:736, 1980.

40. Horrobin, D.; "Gamma-Linolenic Acid in Medicine," *1984–85 Yearbook of Nutiritional Medicine,* J. Bland (ed.), Keats Publishing, Inc., New Canaan, Connecticut, p. 30, 1985.

41. Velardo, B.; et al.; "Decrease of Platelet Activity after Intake of Small Amounts of Eicosapentaenoic Acid in Diabetics," *Throm. Haemostas.* 48(3):344, 1982.

42. Horrobin, D.; "Gamma-Linolenic Acid in Medicine," *1984–85 Yearbook of Nutritional Medicine,* J. Bland (ed.), Keats Publishing, Inc., New Canaan, Connecticut, p. 25, 1985.

43. Smith, D.W.; *Recognizable Patterns of Human Malformation,* 3rd edition, Saunders, Philadelphia, 1982.

44. Clarren, S.K.; Smith, D.W.; "The Fetal Alcohol Syndrome," *New Engl. J. Med.* 198:1063–1067, 1978.

45. Church, M.W.; Gerkin, K.P.; "Hearing Disorders in Children with Fetal Alcohol Syndrome: Findings From Case Reports," *Pediatrics* 82(2): 1988.

46. Ibid.

47. Chandra, R.K.; "Single Nutrient Deficiency and Cell-Mediated Immunity: Zinc," *Amer. J. Clin. Nutr.* 33:736, 1980.

48. Beisel, W.R.; "Single Nutrients and Immunity," *Am. J. Clin. Nutr.* 35(Suppl.):449–451, 1982.

49. Allen, J.; Kay, N.; McClain, C.; "Severe Zinc Deficiency in Humans: Association with T-Lymphocyte Dysfunction," *Ann. Int. Med.* 95:154–7, 1981.

50. Golden, M.; Jackson, A.; Golden, B.; "Effect of Zinc on Thymus of Recently Malnourished Children," *Lancet* ii:1057–9, 1977.

51. Hamblin, J.; Hussain, J.; Akbar, A.; et al.; "Immunological Reason for Chronic Ill Health after Infectious Mononucleosis," *Brit. Med. J.* 287:85–88, 1983.

52. Willmott, F.; Say, J.; Downey, D.; et al.; "Zinc and Recalcitrant Trichomoniasis," *Lancet* i:1053, 1983.

53. Klevay, L.M.; Keck, S.; Bacome, D.F.; "Evidence of Dietary Copper and Zinc Deficiencies," *J.A.M.A.* 241(18):1916–1918, 1979.

54. Chandra, R.K.; "Trace Element Regulation of Immunity and Infection," *J. Am. Coll. Nutr.* 4(1):5–16, 1985.

55. Kiremidjian-Schumacher, L.; Stotzky, G.; "Selenium and Immune Responses," *Environ. Res.* 42:277–303, 1987.

56. Kidd, P.; "Germanium-132: Homeostatic Normalizer and Immunostimulant—A Review of its Preventive and Therapeutic Efficacy," *Intl. Clin. Nutr. Rev.* Special Article 7(1), 1987.

57. Chandra, R.K.; "Nutrition and Immunity—Basic Considerations," Part 1, *Contemp. Nutr.* 11(11), 1986.

58. Wright, J.; Suen, R.M.; *A Human Clinical Study of Ester-C vs. L-Ascorbic Acid*, Meridian Valley Clinical Laboratory, Kent, Washington, 1988.

59. Kaul, T.N.; et al.; "Antiviral Effect of Flavonoids on Human Viruses," *J. Med. Virol.* 15:71–79, 1985.

60. Werbach, M.; *"Nutritional Influences on Illness,"* Third Line Press, Inc., Tarzana, California, p. 259, 1988.

61. Ames, S.R.; "Factors Affecting Absorption, Transport and Storage of Vitamin A," *Am. J. Clin. Nutr.* 22:934, 1969.

62. Tappel, A.L.; *Nutrition Today,* July-Aug., 1973.

63. Prasad, J.S.; "Effect of Vitamin E on Leukocyte Function," *Am. J. Clin. Nutr.* 33:606–8, 1980.

64. Axelrod, A.E.; Traketellis, A.C.; "Relationship of Pyridoxine to

Immunological Phenomena," *Vitam. Horm.* 22:591–607, 1964.

65. Chandra, R.K.; "Nutrition and Immunity—Basic Considerations," Part 1, *Contemp. Nutr.* 11(11), 1986.

66. Levy, J.A.; "Nutrition and the Immune System," in Stites, D.P., et al. *Basic and Clinical Immunology,* fourth edition, Lange Medical Publications, Los Altos, California, pp. 297–305, 1982.

67. Ibid.

68. Beisel, W.R.; Edelman, R.; et al.; "Single Nutrient Effects on Immunologic Function," *J.A.M.A.* 245:53–58, 1981.

69. Das, U.N.; "Antibiotic-Like Action of Fatty Acids," *Can. Med. Assoc. J.* 132:1350, 1985.

70. Bean, W.B.; Hodges, R.E.; Daum, K.; "Pantothenic Acid Deficiency Induced in Human Subjects," *Proc. Soc. Exper. Biol. Med.* 86, 693–698, 1954.

71. Beisel, W.R.; Edelman, R.; et al.; "Single Nutrient Effects on Immunologic Function," *J.A.M.A.* 245:53–58, 1981.

72. Hodges, R.E.; Bean, W.B.; et al.; "Factors Affecting Human Antibody Response," *Am. J. Clin. Nutr.* 11(2):85–93, 1962.

73. Wara, D.W.; Ammann, A.J.; "Thymosin Treatment of Children with Primary Immunodeficiency Disease," *Transpl. Proc.* 10(1):203–209, 1978.

74. Bach, J.F.; "Thymic Hormones," *J. Immunophar.* 1(3):277–310, 1979.

75. Rubenstein, A.; et al.; "In Viro and In Vitro Effects of Thymosin and Adenosine Deaminase on Adenosine-Deaminase-Deficient Lymphocytes,: *New Engl. J. Med.* 300(8):387–392, 1979.

76. Aiuti, F.; et al.; "Thymopoietin Pentapeptide Treatment of Primary Immunodeficiencies," *Lancet* 551–554, 1983.

77. Paul, S.; "The Virus Crisis," Lecture presented in Bloomington Minnesota, Feb. 24, 1990.

Index

Index

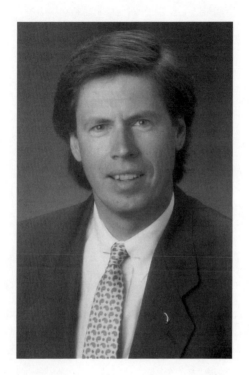

Dr. Michael A. Schmidt is Visiting Professor of Applied Biochemistry and Clinical Nutrition at Northwestern College. He is on the Scientific Council of the International and American Association of Clinical Nutritionists, and is a Scientific Advisor to the International Academy of Nutrition and Preventive Medicine. He is a senior scientist with HealthComm Clinical Research Center in Gig Harbor, Washington. The author of *Beyond Antibiotics* and *Tired of Being Tired*, Dr. Schmidt makes his home in the Puget Sound area of Washington.